HOW TO HEAL ULCERATIVE COLITIS *Naturally*:

A KICK-ASS, Take-Charge Approach!

By A. Ball & G. Ball

Publisher: Ball Media Innovations, Inc.
Pembroke Pines, Florida

For more information visit: https://successfulhealing.com

ISBN – Paperback: 979-8-9905764-0-7

First Edition: May 2024

The information provided by this book is for informational purposes only. It should not be used to diagnose or treat any illness. Therapies discussed in this book potentially carry risks that are undisclosed. All health decisions should be made in conjunction with advice from a qualified healthcare practitioner. While all attempts have been made to verify information provided in this publication, neither the author nor the publisher assumes any responsibility for errors, omissions, or contrary interpretation of the subject matter herein. This publication is not intended for use as a source of legal, medical advice or any other type of professional advice. The information contained herein may be subject to change at any time. The purchaser of this publication assumes responsibility for the use of these materials and information.

Neither the publisher nor the author is engaged in rendering professional advice or services to individual readers. The ideas, procedures, and suggestions in this book are not intended as a substitute for consulting your physician. All matters regarding your health require medical supervision. The author is not a physician or medical professional. Neither the publisher nor the author shall be liable or responsible for any loss or damage allegedly arising from any information or suggestion in this book.

The recipes in this book are to be followed as written. The publisher and author is not responsible for your specific health or allergy needs that may require medical supervision. Neither the author nor the publisher are responsible for any adverse reactions to the recipes, supplements or medications contained in this book.

The author and publisher assume no responsibility or liability whatsoever on the behalf of any purchaser or reader of these materials. Any perceived slights of specific people or organizations are unintentional. Any stated opinions are the author's alone, unless otherwise noted, and do not represent anyone else.

We are not medical doctors and therefore cannot make recommendations that are health related. We are not making any promises or endorsing or condemning any products, businesses, doctors, books, or people.

By reading this book you agree that we are in no way responsible for your choice to participate or not to participate in any mentioned activity, and/or for anything resulting from that choice. We do not guarantee that this book contains the latest information or accurate information. Everything in this book is subject to change, and there may be relevant information not covered here.

We have included information and opinions from medical professionals as well as laypersons. We are not responsible for this information, or their advice and opinions. We do not necessarily agree with every opinion expressed in this book. Do not make choices based on the authority of the material in this book. Everyone is different. What has been safe for us and others mentioned in this book may not have the same effect on you. What feels acceptable to us may feel different to you.

The contents of this book is for informational purposes only. The Content is not intended to be a substitute for professional medical advice. Always seek the advice of your physician or other qualified health provider with any questions you may have regarding a medical condition. Never disregard professional medical advice because of something you have read in this book. We do not recommend or endorse any specific physicians, products, procedures, opinions, or other information that may be mentioned in this book. Reliance on any information provided by this book is solely at your own risk.

This book contains links to various sites. We are not responsible for the content, software, or the privacy practices of such websites. We are not responsible for the products, claims, information or the links to other sites on these sites. The Linked Sites are provided for your convenience only, and you access them at your own risk.

This book mentions a variety of companies. We are not responsible for the products, claims, information or service of those companies. We are not endorsing any companies, services or products. The information on these companies are for your convenience only and you contact and use them at your own risk.

The information and opinions expressed in this book cite our personal experience. Wherever personal opinions and testimonials are expressed, be aware that your experiences will not necessarily be the same.

You are urged to use your own judgment and discretion and to consult with your doctor.

Use of this book signifies your agreement to the above terms.

CONTENTS

We believe that the ability to gather, use and share this information was given to us by the grace of God. Now we share it with you, in the hopes that it will change your life for the better. May God bless you with healing, peace and joy.

FOREWARD

Though this is my wife's story, this is mine also. It was the summer of 2019 and I was sitting in our den watching a New York Mets game when suddenly I heard a blood-curdling scream coming from behind the bathroom door. I jumped to my feet, which was tough because I have an electric recliner chair that unfolds and folds back very slowly. I was out of the chair having never folded it back.

I was about to break down the bathroom door (not sure if I could) when I called out asking "Are you okay?" My wife answered and let me know that the pain was unbearable. She cracked open the door and told me that she was bleeding rectally and had horrible cramps and pain. I saw the blood in the toilet bowl. It was frightening.

This was the start of a period of months with the same screaming, moaning, and crying. What was happening? We contacted our Gastroenterologist and made an appointment.

During his first exam, he mentioned a term I have never heard before... "Ulcerative Colitis". I recognized Colitis because I had professionally edited a video for the Crohn's Colitis Foundation a few years earlier, but I never thought about it again. Now it was something that was taking over our lives.

We scheduled my wife for a colonoscopy, but the doctor suggested that we needed to wait for her bleeding to stop. When it finally slowed down enough, we scheduled the colonoscopy. My wife was wheeled away, and I sat in the waiting room and waited for the doctor to come out.

About 45 minutes later, he came out and told me that my wife was not well. He said that her entire colon was totally inflamed, ulcerated and irritated. Again, he mentioned

Ulcerative Colitis. That day led to a total change in our lives. My wife could not leave our house because of the symptoms, so we mostly stayed inside. We had recently recovered from what we now believe was Covid, so we had already been homebound for quite some time. I work from home, so now I was only left to do errands such as shopping.

During this time, my wife did lots of research, and learned everything she could about UC. She devised her own treatment regimen that seemed to work. Gradually she improved. Though at first, she still had flareups, she never gave up. She was a real trooper! She tweaked her program and ultimately, she was able to conquer all the UC symptoms. As you can imagine, this has been a massive relief for both of us.

There are so many people out there suffering and lost. With all her research and her success, we felt that she could help others. Thus, together, we created this book for you.

Congratulations on purchasing this book. I hope and pray it helps you immensely! Stand strong and don't give up. Make the difficult decisions and choose the things that will help you in the long run. God bless you.

G. Ball

CHAPTER 1: THE STORM OF ULCERATIVE COLITIS

I'm going to tell you a story with a happy ending. I'll share the details of how I went from agony caused by ulcerative colitis to no symptoms of it whatsoever, along with normal test results.

And by the way, in the process, I also cleared up chronic, severe gastritis.

If you've picked up this book, either you or someone you care about was diagnosed with ulcerative colitis or perhaps Crohn's disease. You or they were probably told that there is no cure, and that you'd have to take medication for the rest of your life. And you may have been told that the cause of this disease is unknown.

By the grace of God, I have found that there is hope and help. By addressing potential root causes, I found that the disease can and does reverse.

What I did, you can do also.

These days, rather than remaining passive, it's essential to take charge of your own care. Yes, there's a lot to know, but once you learn, you can steer your own ship in a direction that leads to healing. Even if you have doctors you trust, you'll be more likely to get better care if you learn and participate.

I hope that you will consider this book as a starting point to put together your own program. As I did, you'll want to research, and pick and choose what's best for you, based on your unique situation. I'll share info that can help you get started.

Since being diagnosed with ulcerative colitis, on social media, I've come across thousands who are struggling with this awful disease, and don't know what to do. They don't know that there are natural ways to treat this disease. Or they're seeing only part of what's needed to heal fully. That's why I've written this book.

In my research I found that I couldn't get all the information I needed in one place. I also found that what might have worked for someone else, wasn't right or enough for me. While there are a couple of very expensive programs you can buy into that promise healing from ulcerative colitis, I didn't agree with everything they recommended. Plus, the cost of these programs will mean that many won't be able to afford them.

It's my belief that what worked so well for me can help others. And if your situation is different, you can still use the information in this book to find your own path to healing. And in my heart, it's my desire to give this information to you in an inexpensive and accessible way. I hope it will help you to get your life back.

The program I put together for myself required commitment. It took years to get into this mess, and I had to apply myself to getting well. While it wasn't easy, it was doable, worked amazingly, and in my opinion, it was so worth the effort. Eventually I was able to taper off supplements, broaden my diet, etc. So, everything I had to do for a while wasn't what I had to do forever.

In my research, most of what I did for ulcerative colitis was also showing promise for Crohn's disease. While I don't have direct experience with Crohn's, my guess is that what you see in this book might be just as effective for Crohn's.

For ulcerative colitis, if you're looking for a quick fix or a single pill to take, you won't find that here. If you want to take that path, you may be able to suppress your symptoms, to some extent, with drugs. However, the drugs currently used by the medical community for ulcerative colitis have some serious potential side effects. Some of which might be life span altering. And for many, they don't work all that well.

Check out this quote from a PubMed Central article on the use of bone broth for ulcerative colitis:

"Currently, the drugs used for the treatment of this disease are based on the administration of anti-inflammatory and immunosuppressive drugs for long periods, the disadvantage of these is that they are expensive, and have a low degree of effectiveness, with several side effects, unlike therapies based on a nutritional approach have proven to be effective for the treatment and prevention of chronic diseases, without causing side effects."

More importantly, as I mentioned, the drugs are designed to suppress symptoms. They are not able to fix the root causes of the problem. Yet, ulcerative colitis can steal your life and happiness. For me, I felt something had to be done beyond what I was being offered. It was only logical to try to identify and address the potential root causes of the illness.

On the other hand, concerning how fast one can heal, the gut wall replaces itself every 3-5 days. So, anything is possible if we help create the right environment for the body to heal and restore itself.

You might find my personal program overwhelming. It can also be costly to use various herbs and supplements, get medical testing, and to follow specific diets. Do you need to do all that I did? I don't know.

My feeling is that the strategies I needed are what was necessary for <u>me</u> to heal ulcerative colitis. However, you may not require everything I did. Even some small changes might make a difference for you. What you do is up to you, and I always suggest prayer and asking for God's leading. That's how I roll.

For some of you, finding a good holistic/functional doctor who can guide you will be important. At the very least, you'll want to find one who will be willing to give you the tests I'll be discussing. This can help you identify your own root causes of ulcerative colitis, so that you can address them.

Before I go into the details of what I did, I'll share the start of my experience with ulcerative colitis.

First, I want to remind you that I'm not a doctor. I'm simply a person who did my research and had success. In this book, I will touch on why certain things may have helped me, but as a layperson I'll leave the in-depth medical/technical discussions to others. I'll be writing more from the perspective of sharing what I did, what worked for me, and what didn't. I'll also share potential root causes, some of which I had and some which I didn't have. I'll share info on how to deal with the various root causes. Finally, I'll share information on other things you might want to take a look at that I've found might be helpful, that I didn't do myself.

If this book helps you, that's so awesome, but don't take this as medical advice. Use this book as a start-off for your own research. And again, I'll say that it's important to always consult with your own physician. If you can find a holistic, integrative or functional physician who understands the gut, even better. In fact, much better. Sometimes getting the opinion of multiple types of doctors is helpful as well.

The Beginning of the Problem

In the summer of 2019, it all started unexpectantly — in the dentist's chair. I was having some rather stressful work done when the stomach pain began. Suddenly, in the middle of being worked on by the dentist, uncomfortable spasms seized my abdomen, catching me off guard. I made it through the procedure and got home.

Of course, I wondered why this was happening. I had realized I had some mildly spicey food the day before. I assumed that given the spice along with the stress at the dentist, I was experiencing something that would pass shortly. Unfortunately, this was just the beginning of my unbearable experience with ulcerative colitis.

The Unfolding Nightmare

Within days of my dental appointment, my world turned upside down. What started as some discomfort soon transformed into a torrent of symptoms that would redefine the meaning of agony for me. And I'm a person who has lived with head-to-toe pain due to a variety of chronic and painful health issues.

The first inkling of serious trouble came in the form of rectal bleeding. Within a couple days it began. At first, it was subtle, but it swiftly escalated into non-stop heavy bleeding. I was seeing a lot of bright red blood on the tissue paper, in the bowl and embedded in the feces. Honestly, this was terrifying. My imagination went to work overtime.

Then the stomach pain escalated into intense spasming pain internally, deep in my gut, happening almost constantly. The cramping became so severe that I was literally screaming in agony. It became worse when I ate or when I had bowel movements. My poor husband was listening to me scream in pain day and night.

The next symptom to show up was diarrhea. This turned my life into a relentless sprint to the bathroom. Every 15 minutes to a half hour I had to get to the bathroom. Sometimes there was nothing to release, and sometimes it was liquid.

Even the nights became a marathon of constant bathroom visits. I became more and more exhausted from pain and lack of sleep, which is tough when you already have chronic fatigue and apnea.

At this point, I could no longer leave the house. I always had to be close to the bathroom. I already had a limited lifestyle because of my other health issues. These symptoms caused me to become completely isolated from everyone but my husband. He worked from home and was almost always there. He was wonderfully supportive, but this was tough on him too!

Eating became a paradox—an essential act that morphed into an ordeal. Everything I consumed seemed to provoke my insides, triggering severe cramping and sharp, stabbing pains.

The gastroenterologist told me to go on a liquid diet. I began drinking protein drinks, but the liquids still caused the same excruciating pain.

I found myself caught in a horrible cycle where food, the very source of life, became a source of suffering. Ultimately, I shed over 40 pounds. While I really did need to lose this weight, this was not a weight loss plan I'd recommend to anyone.

The Colonoscopy and results

It took a couple of months before I could get scheduled for a colonoscopy. As I'll discuss later on, a colonoscopy is the best way for doctors to see what's actually happening in the gut. It allows them to identify issues, take a biopsy, if necessary, remove polyps, etc. The doctor preferred not to go inside when I was bleeding because it could be easier to perforate the bowel. We were giving it time to see if it would stop. However, the bleeding was not stopping.

To help with symptoms during the wait, my gastroenterologist was on vacation and another gastro in his office recommended an over-the-counter product you can find in pharmacies called IBgard. It's made with peppermint oil and is supposed to help with cramping, bowel urgency, diarrhea, gas, etc. I was excited to try something natural. Unfortunately, I developed chest pain and a rapid heartbeat. We ended up calling 911 and I had a ride to the emergency room. I was fine, but there was no way I was taking that again.

I found a few things did work, though slightly. I drank peppermint tea, which I found soothing. Bigalow tea bags were gluten free, and I went through a lot of them. I also drank marshmallow root tea quite a lot, which I bought in bulk from my local health food store. This was also somewhat soothing. I took slippery elm capsules for its ability to create mucus, which in turn can help protect the gastrointestinal tract. Again, slightly soothing.

Prior to the procedure, I finally slowed the bleeding down by fasting for 10 days, with nothing but water, bone broth and medicinal manuka honey. I'll talk about that in detail later. While it didn't stop the bleeding 100%, it did diminish it quite a bit.

I had the colonoscopy in September of 2019. When they finally looked inside, the doctor came to give my husband and I the news. He said it didn't look good and there was some difficult news.

I had pancolitis – ulcerative colitis throughout my entire colon.

Where do I go from here?

While waiting for my doctor's recommendations, I researched the drugs being used to manage ulcerative colitis. Not one was a cure. Every one of them had severe potential side effects. Some were potentially life shortening.

When I saw my doctor, his only recommendation was to go on the drug Mesalamine. It would cost me hundreds of dollars a month and would reduce the inflammation. I was told that it would not heal ulcerative colitis, but it would just suppress the symptoms.

I looked into the side effects that this drug was known to have, and the potential long-term damage it could do. While I would have taken it if there was nothing else I could do, I did not want to go on it if there was an alternative. According to my doctor, there was not.

Yet, throughout my entire adult life, I had often used alternatives to handle various illnesses. Because of certain genetic predispositions, I often tended to struggle with drug side effects. So, I found that I usually did better using herbs, supplements, minerals and diet along with various alternative treatments. While it was not always possible to successfully deal with every illness this way, I found that it often was.

Before I developed ulcerative colitis, I had been diagnosed with a number of difficult chronic health issues over my life, including late-stage Lyme disease, chronic fatigue, fibromyalgia, environmental illness and immune disorders. By necessity, I had already learned a great deal about alternative health methods.

After more than 40 years of learning and applying holistic health methods to myself (and my husband too), I knew quite a bit by the time ulcerative colitis showed up. As a layperson, I was experienced with the use of herbs, vitamins, and minerals to create healing and balance in the body. Most of all, I knew how to research. I've been asked more times than I could count whether I was a doctor. Of course, the answer was and is no. I am not a doctor. I'm just someone who has had to learn in order to stay alive.

By this time, I believed in the holistic philosophy of health:

Find and heal the root cause of the illness, if possible.

What could be smarter than that? Granted, as I said above, sometimes it's not possible. But often it is.

Then there was the addition of my own personal philosophy of healing:

Treat with the least invasive approaches and use whatever will work that offers the least side effects.

So, I had a history to fall back on, and over the years, I had experienced success with many issues. For example, I had dissolved gallstones when most doctors would have simply removed the gallbladder. I had before and after ultrasounds to prove it.

Also, I had healed various infections without prescription antibiotics. Some were very severe such as bronchitis, or an infected spider bite that swelled my thigh up massively and was weeping pus. It was completely healed, using alternatives rather than pharmaceutical antibiotics.

I knew I had managed various other health issues without the use of drugs. I was determined to see if I could do the same with ulcerative colitis. If it was possible to heal ulcerative colitis without the use of drugs, I wanted to know. At the very least, I wanted to minimize the use of pharmaceutical drugs.

I started my research with my gastroenterologist. I mentioned to my doctor that I'd like to try a natural route. I was hoping he'd share what he knew about this type of health support with me. Instead, he literally laughed at me, saying it was impossible.

Next, I reached out to various doctors and health industry professionals, read every book I could find, joined a lot of relevant social media groups, perused medical studies, and just searched, searched, searched for anything relevant. Gradually, I put together my own plan, and gradually I healed.

Months later my gastroenterologist who had laughed at me would reverse his position, saying that he couldn't argue with success. I hoped he'd take my experience and share it with his patients. I tried to share my process with him, and he was polite but uninterested in what I did to get well.

So, I'll go into the details of exactly what I did to obtain that success with you.

And of course, all the glory goes to God, who helped me, led me and loved me throughout this situation. I feel it's God who has encouraged me to write this book, hopefully to help you, who He loves.

Chapter 1: The Storm of Ulcerative Colitis

CHAPTER 2: WHAT IS ULCERATIVE COLITIS?

Let's take a minute to look at the disease. Ulcerative colitis (UC) is a member of the inflammatory bowel disease (IBD) family, causing inflammation and ulcers specifically in the colon and rectum. It's miserable.

UC is different from Crohn's, which can take up ground throughout your digestive tract. Although I haven't had the experience of treating Crohn's, my guess is that what I did for UC could also help with Chron's.

Ulcerative colitis is usually diagnosed by a colonoscopy which enables your doctor to see the colon. It is not identifiable through a blood test. I tend to stay away from anything that's invasive, but this is one invasive test I felt was necessary. In my opinion, it's important to rule out cancer, to remove any pre-cancerous polyps, and to get an accurate diagnosis. A colonoscopy allows for this.

For those who are scared, I'd say that the experience of the procedure was very tolerable. In fact, not at all uncomfortable. I had an endoscopy at the same time, which allows the doctor to check the upper GI tract, including the esophagus, stomach and the first part of the small intestine. As you are knocked out during the experience, neither procedure left me with any additional pain or discomfort.

The most challenging part is how you're required to prepare. There's fasting involved and something you take to clean out your bowels that keeps you running to the bathroom. Not fun but tolerable.

Years ago, I had gone through a colonoscopy and the prep had caused me to lose electrolytes. I had high blood pressure and an irregular heartbeat. This time I purchased an electrolyte replenishment product with the approval of my doctor. I took that while I was prepping for the procedure. I did much better. It was important to find something that was gluten free, and free of any irritants, coloring, etc. I used a product called elete Electrolyte which you can add to water or any other drink.

Symptoms of Ulcerative Colitis

Although there can be different degrees of symptoms, the more common symptoms of ulcerative colitis can include:

Abdominal Discomfort: Cramps and pain in the abdomen which can range from mild or severe.

For me, pain was at 11 on a scale of 1 to 10. I found myself screaming in pain a lot. I've never had a child, but I've heard this pain compared to being in labor. I don't know if it's true, but it sure seemed like it might be similar.

Frequent Bathroom Timeouts: UC can disrupt your regular life with urgency and increased frequency of bowel movements. There can also be an almost constant sense of urgency even though your bowels are empty. I experienced this nonstop for months.

Bleeding: Blood can show up in the stool. It usually comes from ulcers that are in the large intestine or rectum. There can also be pus and mucus in the stools.

How the blood appears can indicate what's going on inside. Bright red blood can often come from the lower gastrointestinal tract, closer to the anus or rectum. It can be from hemorrhoids, anal fissures or from bleeding in the lower colon. Dark and tarry stools may mean bleeding higher up in the gastrointestinal tract such as in the stomach or upper small intestine.

If the blood appears to be mixed in with the stool, it could be coming from the colon or rectum. Ulcerative colitis,

Crohn's or polyps could be a possible cause. Blood clots or mucus can suggest inflammation in the tract as with colitis.

Diarrhea: This can be occasional or a few episodes, or it can be frequent. For me, it was non-stop for months. Diarrhea can cause depletion in minerals so if this is a symptom, it's important to replenish electrolytes, but be careful to replenish with a product that won't be irritating to the gut. As I mentioned above, I purchased a product called elete Electrolyte that I used for the colonoscopy preparation. It was also helpful while I was experiencing diarrhea.

Fever. This is usually chronic and low grade. I consistently ran just over 99.

Weight Loss: In addition to the discomfort associated with eating causing a reduction in food intake, UC can affect your body's ability to absorb nutrients. All of this can cause weight loss.

Fatigue: UC doesn't limit its impact to the gut; it can also drain your energy reserves, leaving you feeling fatigued and worn out. I found that I was up much of the night using the bathroom because of the ulcerative colitis. Sleep was difficult anyway with the level of pain. Plus, I was becoming vitamin deficient from being unable to eat much at all. I believe this all contributed to a heavy-duty fatigue.

Nausea: Some people wrestle with queasiness or outright nausea. The things I'd commonly took for nausea were irritating to my gut, including sugary ginger and ginger ale. I really didn't find an ideal way to treat the nausea initially, but ultimately everything I did in my personal program removed that issue.

While there are other possible symptoms, these are the most common. Personally, I had them all, and severely.

Chapter 2: What is Ulcerative Colitis?

CHAPTER 3: UNRAVELING POSSIBLE CAUSES OF ULCERATIVE COLITIS

Ulcerative colitis is a bit of a puzzle. For some people, the cause can be tracked down to a single issue such as a bacterial or parasitic infection. For others, it can be more complex. I'm not sure that all of the possible root causes have been identified, but let's talk about some of the potential causes that are known.

Genetic Threads in the Tapestry

One significant thread in the intricate tapestry of ulcerative colitis lies within the realm of genetics. Family history correlates with a heightened risk for those who have relatives grappling with inflammatory bowel diseases. Genetic markers, though not deterministic, hint at a hereditary component.

According to Medline Plus, these genetic markers can indicate a predisposition to autoimmune issues. This causes the body to have an abnormal immune response to normal bacteria in the digestive tract. It attacks itself. The variations can also cause changes in the intestinal lining's protective function.

Medline Plus also says the following:

> *"The inner surface of the intestines provides a barrier that protects the body's tissues from the bacteria that live in the intestines and from toxins that pass through the digestive tract. Researchers speculate that a breakdown of this barrier allows contact between the intestinal tissue and the bacteria and toxins, which can trigger an immune reaction. This immune response may lead to chronic inflammation and the digestive problems characteristic of ulcerative colitis."*

Apparently, this can be caused by genetics.

My mother had bleeding ulcers when I was in my teens. While I understand that this means there was an increased likelihood of UC, I don't believe that this means it's inevitable. I would say that with a family history of UC, it's a good idea to take preventative precautions. Many physicians believe that genetic predispositions don't have to be expressed if we give our bodies what they need to thrive.

Immunological Challenges

As mentioned in the genetic section, a problem with the immune system, our body's guardian, can be a root cause of ulcerative colitis. Gone rogue, it can target the delicate lining of the colon. This is called autoimmune disease. The big question is why did it go rogue! Why does the immune system perceive something of its own as a threat?

The bigger question is this: Can it be stopped without taking immune suppressants? Immune suppressants can cause all kinds of serious problems.

Many functional doctors have had success reversing autoimmune diseases, and in my program, I implemented some of the strategies they use. Those will be coming up in future chapters.

Environmental Influences

With ulcerative colitis, external factors can feed the fire. This could include issues ranging from dietary habits to exposure to certain microbes or parasites. It can include air pollution, and certain drugs.

Even mold exposure can be a possible cause. Combine mold exposure with a genetic predisposition to inflammatory bowel disease and you have the components needed to create UC.

An article on the Sponaugle Wellness Institute site states the following:

> *"A study published in the Journal of Environmental and Public Health found that there was a link between mold exposure and gastrointestinal issues, including inflammatory bowel disease such as ulcerative colitis. The study also found that individuals who were genetically susceptible to inflammatory bowel disease were more likely to develop symptoms after mold exposure."*

Ultimately, healing or improvement for some people can be a matter of cleaning up these things in a health supporting manner. My theory was that if I could get rid of these burdens on my body, it could reverse the symptoms of ulcerative colitis.

Gut Microbiota - A Balancing Act

Within our digestive system lies a massive community of microorganisms, collectively known as the gut microbiota, or microbiome. Within this community, there's a delicate balance between beneficial and harmful microbes. A healthy balance will maintain the equilibrium of gut health. Yet, disruptions to this equilibrium may tip the scales towards inflammation, and ultimately UC.

Drugs can impact the gut microbiome. For example, a round of antibiotics can change everything. It kills the good with the bad. Restoring equilibrium can help heal the digestive system.

Infection

As mentioned above, a possible cause might be an untreated bacterial, parasitic, or fungal infection. Even viral infections are thought to be a possible cause. These can contribute to the development of ulcerative colitis. Even after killing these infections, for some people, the body might continue inappropriately creating an immune response of inflammation. So once the infection has been treated, it's still possible to develop UC. However, I believe that it's possible to calm down inappropriate immune reactions naturally, and to calm inflammation naturally.

Stress

Life's tribulations, both big and small, can leave a mark on our well-being. Stress is thought to be another potential contributor to the development of ulcerative colitis. While it's usually not thought of as the total cause, the intricate interplay between our mental state and the delicate balance within the gut may be as important to look at as the previous factors. We'll talk about that in more depth later on.

Unhealthy diet

In my opinion, if your gastroenterologist tells you that diet has nothing to do with getting ulcerative colitis, and with treating it, he/she would be wrong. Yet, that's what a lot of doctors will tell their patients.

While I'm not sure that poor diet alone could cause UC, I believe it can be a part of what leads to it. And changing the diet can be a huge part of a recovery plan. It's only common sense.

Everyone knows that diet impacts the microbiome, and that a healthy microbiome is essential to good gut health. Research has shown that the gut microbiome plays a role in regulating the immune system and maintaining the integrity of the intestinal barrier. When there is an imbalance in the microbiome, it can potentially lead to an inappropriate immune response and inflammation in the gut, contributing to conditions like ulcerative colitis.

To say that diet doesn't matter is refusing to look at the obvious. Diet matters to the gut and to overall health. In fact, I would go so far as to say that a change in diet will be one of the most important things you can do to get well.

So, if you've been eating things like processed foods, lots of sugar (real or sugar substitutes) and simple carbs, unhealthy fats, not enough veggies, inflammatory foods, and other things that your particular body doesn't like, that may have contributed to your situation.

Other Considerations: Celiac & Gluten Intolerance

These are conditions that don't necessarily cause ulcerative colitis. However, they might relate to the development, or predispose someone to get it.

Consider that the composition of gluten in grains has changed over time, particularly with the development of modern wheat varieties through agricultural practices and breeding. The gluten found in contemporary wheat and other grains differs from that in ancient or heirloom varieties. This may be why so many people have problems digesting it.

Over the years, traditional wheat varieties have undergone hybridization and selective breeding to improve traits such as yield, disease resistance, and baking qualities. While these efforts have been successful in enhancing certain aspects of wheat, they have also led to changes in the gluten protein composition.

Modern wheat varieties often contain higher levels of gluten proteins, particularly the gliadin component. Gliadins are one of the gluten protein groups associated with gluten-related disorders.

Also, some concerns have been raised about the potential impact of glyphosate, a widely used herbicide, on wheat crops. Glyphosate residue may be present in conventionally grown wheat, and studies have suggested possible associations with gluten-related disorders.

All of these changes in gluten can have implications for individuals with gluten-related issues.

According to the Celiac Disease Foundation, celiac disease is an autoimmune disease that occurs in genetically predisposed people. When people with celiac disease eat gluten, the body mounts an immune response that attacks the small intestine. While celiac does not cause ulcerative colitis, those with celiac have an increased incidence of Crohn's and ulcerative colitis.

If you have untreated celiac, it can impact your overall health. Untreated celiac disease is associated with an increased risk of developing other autoimmune disorders, such as ulcerative colitis, type 1 diabetes, thyroid disorders, and autoimmune liver diseases. It can increase the risk of cancer, and it can cause gastrointestinal complications like lactose intolerance, gallbladder dysfunction, and an increased risk of gastrointestinal cancers. A simple blood test can identify celiac disease.

Gluten intolerance is a different possibility.

It's not an autoimmune response, but it is a cause of digestive issues for many people. It can be diagnosed due to digestive symptoms and reactions to gluten.

One way to test would be to abstain from any gluten containing foods for several weeks to months, to see if you feel better. You can choose to reintroduce gluten to see if there are any symptoms.

Years before I developed ulcerative colitis, I was diagnosed as gluten intolerant. When I decided to go on a gluten-free diet, I decided to go all the way. I chose to change everything that went in my mouth including medications, toothpaste, and even shampoo and soap which could make its way to my lips. It did make a difference for me for many years.

If I accidentally got "glutened", I'd suffer severely for days. It wouldn't start immediately. It would be apparent 2-3 days later. I'd experience increased pain throughout my body, increased fatigue, and the feeling of being sick and feverish. It would also impact my mood with depression.

As I worked on healing from ulcerative colitis, I continued to make sure that everything that went into my mouth was gluten free. Surprisingly, gluten can be found in so many unexpected places. Even spices that you buy in the grocery store can have gluten in them.

Thankfully, since I started eating gluten-free, there are so many more products out there that are being made and marketed. Even some restaurants cater to the gluten-free crowd, such as Outback Steakhouse, Chipotle Mexican Grill and Bolay.

While gluten intolerance may not be the complete cause of ulcerative colitis, I feel that it's essential to deal with it in order to calm the body and the inflammation.

I wonder how many people are gluten intolerant or maybe even have celiac disease, but don't know it!

Chapter 3: Unraveling Possible Causes of Ulcerative Colitis

CHAPTER 4: CONSTRUCTING A PLAN

Prayerfully, I began research. I found everything I could on ulcerative colitis. I ordered and read books, found relevant studies online, watched YouTube videos from doctors and laypeople, studied relevant websites, studied a couple of high-priced courses that were supposed to have the answers, and I consulted with various integrative/functional doctors. (Quite honestly, I found I knew more than some of them who were charging an arm and a leg for consultation fees.)

Little by little I put together my plan.

As I wrote earlier, the gut is a huge part of the immune system. My thinking was that even if this problem was caused by an autoimmune disease, by giving the gut what it needed to heal, reducing inflammation, and by reestablishing proper flora, it could help my immune system work more appropriately. After all, the microbiome in the gut is a known to be a huge part of the immune system.

To accomplish this gut repair, I had certain goals:

- Kill any parasites, excess fungus or bad bacteria overgrowth.
- Stop inflammation.
- Rebuild the lining of the gut.
- Balance the gut flora with the good stuff.
- Support the digestive process.
- Support the immune system.
- Reduce stress.
- Use everything I could find that helps the gut!

Ultimately it worked. I started seeing improvements within a couple weeks, and within a couple months I started seeing major changes. After a couple months, I had a normal fecal test called the calprotectin test. This meant I was not showing inflammation in my gut. We'll talk more about this test, coming up.

Still, it took longer for all of the pain to leave and for the bleeding to stop completely and permanently. Though pain became far less severe within 2-3 months, it only completely left after a couple years. During that time, it was occasional and very mild. After a couple years, there was no more pain or other ulcerative colitis symptoms. I was also free of gastritis symptoms.

The bleeding stopped after a few months but returned a couple times within the first year. One time was when I tried to introduce coffee back to my diet. Ultimately that took a couple years to get to successfully, and now I can drink and enjoy coffee with no ulcerative colitis symptoms or problems. When drinking it at home, I do drop a pinch of baking soda into it to keep it alkaline, but I can enjoy a cup of Starbucks or Dunkin when I'm out, without the baking soda.

I stuck rigidly to the diets I had gone on for 3 years, which I'll go into in future chapters. During that time, I was able to add back in foods which were allowed on the Specific Carbohydrate Diet, and which I tested not to have allergies or sensitivities to.

By the end of the third year, my ulcerative colitis symptoms were long gone, and I was so tired of the limited diet that I finally decided to broaden it. I was able to add back in a number of foods that were off of my diet including some grains, soy, chocolate, tomatoes, potatoes, etc.

I had tested gluten intolerant many years ago and was on a gluten free diet when I developed UC. Though I still remain strictly gluten free, and I monitor and eliminate foods that I show allergies and sensitivities to, I'm not on such a rigid diet any longer.

Also, I've also been able to stop taking most of the supplements I was on specifically for ulcerative colitis. I continue to take probiotics and Boswellia. I'll discuss all the details I just mentioned, coming up.

That said, I have recently loosely gone back on the Paleo Autoimmune diet and the SCD diet for other health issues. Honestly, my other health issues were improved by those diets. I'm choosing to follow those diets, though not as strictly as I was when healing ulcerative colitis. Though my labs continue to show that the inflammation in my gut is within normal limits, in my experience these diets can help body wide.

Let's talk about what I did to get healed.

My Personal Plan

The following pages are the things I did for myself. I will also share about some strategies which for various reasons I was unable to do which might be worth considering.

Following my plan, I was able to get rid of all ulcerative colitis symptoms. This included inflammation in my colon.

So, let's talk about testing.

CHAPTER 5: TESTS YOUR DOCTOR PROBABLY DIDN'T ORDER

There are tests your doctor most likely didn't order for you that I've found really helped me create a targeted treatment for myself.

If you have a mainstream doctor rather than a doctor who slants holistic or functional, there are several tests that you are unlikely to have administered. These tests can give insight into what's happening in your body, and with the guidance of a functional/holistic doctor, they can help with strategy.

I can't stress this enough. It's important to identify what's happening in your body. There may be needs you have that are not addressed in my own personal plan. Testing allows you to tailor your plan to your own needs.

Some of the labs I'll discuss are tests that most mainstream allopathic type doctors don't ordinarily use, even gastroenterologists. And in fact, they may even pooh-pooh these tests, as my gastro did. Even if they're open minded and order some of these tests for you, they probably won't know what to do with the results.

I've found that you'd need a functional/holistic type doctor who knows how to interpret the results, and who knows how to treat you once the results are in. That means finding a savvy functional or holistic doctor who has studied these tests, who understands its interpretation and knows how to treat you based on the results.

If you don't have a doctor like this, you may wish to contact one of the labs I'll mention. They might be able to help you find local doctors who regularly prescribe their tests.

Here are some tests that I've found to be extremely helpful.

Helpful Labs & Tests

Gut Function & Dysbiosis Testing

Your doctor should test you for parasites, fungal infection, bacterial infection and gut functioning.

My gastroenterologist tested me for a few of the more common types of bacteria and parasites in my gut. I came up negative. However, from prior research into this topic, I knew that false negatives are common, especially with parasites. I also knew I was only being tested for a small number of specific bugs.

Finally, I knew there were far more informative tests that could shed light on what was going on in my digestive process. For these, I had to go to my functional/holistic doctor and request them.

One lab that is known for its in-depth gut health tests is Genova Diagnostics. Here's their website address:

https://www.gdx.net/

Their fecal test can give you a wealth of information. Their GI Effects Comprehensive Stool Profile gives you a look inside to see what your digestive function is like. It also gives information on intestinal inflammation, and the intestinal microbiome.

Specifically, it can tell you what fungus, bacteria and parasites are present in your colon, whether or not their numbers are in a healthy range, and whether you're missing any good bacteria.

It can identify how your digestive process is working on many levels. For example, it can tell you if you need to supplement with additional digestive enzymes when you eat, if your acid is low, etc.

With all that information, you can make choices to supplement in order to improve function, to balance the microbiome, to determine whether you have an overgrowth or parasites that require killing, and whether to include other supplements to heal the gut.

Another lab test to consider is the GI-MAP (GI Microbial Assay Plus) by Diagnostic Solutions. They also have a very comprehensive stool analysis. Here's the web address:

https://www.diagnosticsolutionslab.com/tests/gi-map

Nutrient status Test

Another test Genova Diagnostics offers is the NutrEval.

This test lets you know what vitamins you're lacking in so that you can supplement properly to assist your body's healing. It determines the need for antioxidants, vitamins, minerals, amino acids, and fatty acids. It also assesses toxic exposure, which can be an important piece of knowledge to have.

In the beginning when I was experiencing ulcerative colitis full force, I don't think I could have handled a lot of supplements. I had to pick what was the most essential for me personally. This test can help with that.

Mycotoxin from Mold Exposure Test

If there's a possibility that you've been exposed to toxic mold, it can help to have a mycotoxin test to see if you have toxins in your body.

RealTime Laboratories offers a mycotoxin test designed to detect 16 different mycotoxins. You can find information about their test here:

https://realtimelab.com/mycotoxin-testing/

If you suspect you've had exposure to mold, it's important to find and remediate the source of the problem. In fact, it's essential. I've always heard that it's impossible to recover from illness when you're constantly being exposed to toxic mold.

Mold testing companies will come and check your home. We had had and remediated a mold issue in our bathroom years before I got UC. We showed mycotoxins in our tests after that, but we treated to remove them. I'll discuss that in more depth later on.

We periodically retest our home. The mold testing company goes through the entire house, looking for any unwanted moisture. They test the air for spores in all the rooms of our home. Thankfully there were no problems at the time I contracted UC. It can be a big undertaking to fix these types of problems. Plus, it can be expensive.

Allergy & Sensitivity Testing

Food allergies and sensitivities can cause inflammation in the gut. If you can identify the culprits and remove them, you're reducing the stress on your digestive system. Allergies cause reactions pretty much instantly. Sensitivities are similar to allergies only they can take 2-3 days to cause reactions. I felt it was important to identify anything and everything that could irritate the gut and reverse it.

I actually got well before testing for sensitivities. There were some foods that I was surprised to see on the sensitivity list including pineapple, avocado, and dill. I was eating a lot of these, and still got well. These foods are allowed and encouraged on the diets I was following. Still, I think it's helpful to identify what your body is struggling with. Over time, my goal was to repair the gut so that I no longer had allergies or sensitivities.

I'm currently only showing one allergy – eggs. I lost all other food allergies. I'm no longer allergic or even sensitive to dairy. I do still show some food sensitivities and it seems to be around foods that I eat every day. Rotating foods is something that could help with avoiding that, but frankly that's beyond what I've been willing to do. Regardless, I do try to diminish anything I've shown sensitivity to, and I retest periodically.

Calprotectin Test

This is a test that shows whether there's bowel inflammation or not. I didn't receive this test from my doctor right away. He prescribed it one year after my colonoscopy to see if I was making progress. When it came back low normal, he let me know that I would not need another colonoscopy. He felt that this test was an excellent indication of whether or not I was having ulcerative colitis flares and inflammation.

Since I started this program, I've retested Calprotectin at least four times a year. The normal range goes up to a score of 50. My calprotectin scores stayed below 5 while I was on the diets and supplements in my plan. When I broadened my diet to include things such as chocolate, beans, nuts, etc., and went off of some of the supplements, my score crept upwards, up to the 30's and 40's, but still in normal range.

I have found it important to test regularly to see if the changes I was implementing made a difference. This test has been enormously helpful.

Testing for Celiac Disease

As discussed in the prior chapter, celiac is not necessarily a cause of ulcerative colitis, but it can contribute to digestive problems. If anyone has celiac disease, it's important to identify and treat it. Your doctor can order blood work which can identify the presence of antibodies.

Chapter 5: Tests Your Doctor Probably Didn't Order

CHAPTER 6: PARTIAL FASTING TO REST THE DIGESTIVE SYSTEM

To rest my gut, the first thing I did was a partial fast for approximately 10 days. During this time, I cooked and ate only bone broth, and raw manuka honey.

I'm not going to tell you it wasn't difficult. It was. However, I was determined to stop the bleeding. I felt this would help, and it did. Around the 10th day, although not completely stopped, the bleeding slowed down significantly.

Bone Broth

During the fast, I chose to use bone broth because of its amazing properties. It has a number of things in it that can help heal the gut. That includes gelatin, collagen, glycine, trace minerals, amino acids and glutamine.

These things can calm the inflammation and help rebuild the lining of the gut.

According to studies on bone broth, it can act as an anti-inflammatory, decreasing the expression of pro-inflammatory cytokines, and stimulating expression of anti-inflammatory cytokines. All while providing the body with materials that can repair the mucosal lining and reduce ulcerative colitis symptoms.

The one drawback is that bone broth is a high histamine food. There are those who have issues with ingesting high histamine levels. The longer a food is cooked or is kept before eating, the more the histamine content. To minimize this, I cooked the broth for around 24 hours, and used it up quickly. Most of the time I made a new batch every couple of days.

Personally, I'm not a cook and I was in no condition to cook. Regardless, I felt it was essential to make my own bone broth. I had looked into the store-bought versions, and they all had ingredients that I felt could be irritating to my gut such as garlic and onion. And naturally, they were likely to have higher histamine levels.

I invested in a slow cooker and had my husband shop for the ingredients for me. Although bone broth can be made with beef or chicken, I preferred chicken.

I used my mother's chicken soup recipe, minus some ingredients that didn't fit with the diets we'll discuss later. I kept it very simple.

I added one extra ingredient, apple cider vinegar, which draws the healing stuff out of the bones. I kept all the ingredients organic to lower the load on my body.

Here's my basic bone broth soup recipe:

In the slow cooker I added:

8-12 organic, free-range chicken legs. You could use a whole chicken if you prefer, but I chose legs for the bones.

Optional: You can also add some chicken feet if you can get them. Chicken feet are packed with collagen. You can also include other bony parts of the chicken like the neck.

You can also choose beef bones rather than chicken. Be sure to use organic, pasture raised and grass fed if at all possible.

3-4 large organic carrots, washed. If you're eating them directly from the soup, or you'll be blending them to eat, you may wish to chop them into bite size carrot pieces. In the beginning when I was just drinking the broth and throwing away the rest, I just dropped them in whole, or I cut them into several pieces.

3-4 organic celery sticks. I handled these the same as the carrots above, depending on what I'd be doing with them.

Fresh organic dill (you decide how much you like. I used a lot.)

1/2 bunch of fresh organic parsley (to taste, not chopped)

1 tablespoon of the organic apple cider vinegar (I used Bragg Apple Cider Vinegar which was gluten free)

Filtered water to fill the slow cooker after everything else has been added.

Salt to taste. For salt, you can add it to the mix up front, or you can add it to your soup when you're ready to eat. I always use a good quality salt such as a Himalayan salt or Redmond Real Salt. There are those who believe that salt can cause gut problems. I did not find that, but then I didn't use regular table salt.

I let this cook on the highest heat in the slow cooker for about 4 hours, and then I'd lower the heat to a medium setting for another 20 hours. You can go longer if you wish. The settings you use may depend on your slow cooker. The ideal temperature for cooking bone broth is about 180 degrees Fahrenheit.

If you or someone in your household wants the chicken meat, you can remove it from the bones after 4 hours. Then continue cooking the bones and other ingredients. Or you can leave the meat in there. It becomes very tender.

When finished, during the fast I'd strain out all the ingredients. I was left with a simple broth. I drank this for breakfast, lunch and dinner, and whenever the hunger was too much to handle.

Eventually, when I reintroduced solid foods, I ate the chicken and vegetables. I would just remove the skin and bones. At first, I blended the vegetables to make them easier to digest. Eventually when I was ready to move forward, I ate them in their chopped form.

I cooked and ate this soup regularly, for a couple years.

Store this in airtight containers or freeze if you're not going to use it within the next couple of days.

Manuka honey

This rather expensive type of honey is known to have antibacterial properties, including against h. pylori, and staphylococcus aureus (MRSA). I chose to use it while on this fast to manage hunger and to help kill some possible unwanted gut flora. If you have blood sugar issues such as diabetes, I'd run it by your doctor first as it is naturally sweet.

After doing a lot of research on manuka honey and what to get for health purposes, I purchased Manukora UMF 20+/MGO 830+ Raw Manuka Honey on Amazon.com. It's quite expensive, but while I can't prove it, I felt it was worth the investment as part of the whole process.

The UMF and MGO reflect the quality of the honey and this product had the minimum ratings I was looking for. This is one of those times where I won't go into the technical aspect of the product, but it's easy to find on google if you'd like a deeper understanding of manuka honey and how it can help.

Intermittent fasting

Some time ago, I read a book called The Obesity Code: Unlocking the Secrets of Weight Loss by Jason Fung MD. This book gave compelling information on the benefits of fasting for part of the day. While the focus of the book was weight loss and the metabolic system, it occurred to me that this type of fasting would allow my body to rest part of the day. I did see a study indicating that intermittent fasting reduced the inflammatory response in a patient with ulcerative colitis. Since inflammation reduction is the goal, I felt this would fit in with my plan.

As a part of my healing strategy, I would fast from 12-16 hours a day, periodically, so in each 24-hour period I'd only eat during the rest of that window. I didn't do it every day. Sometimes it wasn't practical, and sometimes I just didn't feel that I could handle it. I did it as often as possible, and I continue to do it for the health benefits. I do feel it contributed to my recovery.

Chapter 6: Partial Fasting to Rest the Digestive System

CHAPTER 7: SPECIAL DIETS I WENT ON (AND DIDN'T GO ON)

This is where I took some radical steps. After fasting, I moved onto the next phase, which included some strict diets.

When my symptoms first started, my doctors, including my integrative doctors, suggested certain foods. As I mentioned, eating caused hellish pain in my gut, and they were trying to help. Looking back, I see that all the recommendations were counterproductive.

At one point my gastro recommended I go on a liquid diet. According to him, it didn't matter what kind of liquid I drank, as long as it was liquid. I drank gluten free protein drinks, but this did not help. The liquid caused pain going down, and staying on this liquid diet didn't seem to improve the situation.

All my doctors, including my holistic doctors, recommended a low-residue diet which included a lot of refined carbs such as:

- White bread
- White rice
- Cooked cereals like farina, cream of wheat and grits
- Cold cereals like puffed rice or corn flakes
- Baked potatoes without skin
- Tomato sauce
- Crackers
- Pasta
- Eggs
- Lean meat and fish
- Some fresh fruits and vegetables (with no seeds)
- Dairy (in moderation)

Some of this felt less painful going down such as baked potato. However, I was not making any progress. The pain was severe, I continued to have diarrhea and I bled heavily.

I started researching myself, and found multiple diets linked with calming gut inflammation. In a way, these diets were counter intuitive. I tolerated eating foods such as potatoes and gluten-free white bread better than most other foods, but these would be off-limits on the new diets. Yet, the theory behind these other diets seemed sound and logical. And there's no denying that they were helping people recover from serious health conditions including ulcerative colitis.

Here's what I did.

I went on two different diets and only ate the foods that were accepted on both of them. I also implemented elements of a third and fourth diet. The two main diets were:

- The Specific Carbohydrate Diet or SCD
- Paleo Autoimmune (also referred to as the AIP diet)

The third and fourth diets I used elements of are:

- The Low FODMAP Diet
- The Maker's Diet

Honestly, sticking to these diets was the most challenging part of what I did. As I've mentioned, I don't cook much. In part that's due to issues with pain and fatigue from injuries, CFS and fibromyalgia. In part it's because I don't like to cook, and I never really learned how to cook past the basics. Combine that with the agony I was in with ulcerative colitis, and you know I really didn't want to cook.

Yet, with these diets, I had to cook, no matter how I felt. The only respite I had was when my husband sometimes chipped in and cooked for me, but he was very busy with his business, and didn't like to cook either. So, I had to do whatever it took, keeping it to the minimum necessary.

Also, these diets cut out a lot of the foods I most enjoy. Even though I was eating gluten free when I got ill, I enjoyed my gluten free pasta, breads, cookies, ice cream, etc. Yet, my gut told me (pun intended), it was time to buckle down and do this difficult thing. I needed to treat food as a healing tool. There's that old saying: Do you live to eat or eat to live?

After researching, I felt there was no way around it. If I wanted to remove the inflammation that was causing UC, and heal the gut, I had to do this. I had to eat to live.

Before I go into these diets, I'll share what I chose not to do with my diet, which is to eat vegan.

Some people recommend coming off all animal-based foods, and I saw that there was some short-term help in that for some people. However, through my research, the people I saw making the most progress all seemed to be including animal-based proteins.

In my past, I had followed a vegan diet for a couple years. I became extremely vitamin deficient despite the fact that I studied proper food balancing for vegans. In just this past year, I tried it again for the purpose of losing weight. My hair started falling out, and other worrisome symptoms appeared. I've decided that a vegan diet is not appropriate for me. I'm not sure it's the best option for anyone, but I'm aware that there are studies showing that there are some illnesses it can help with, at least in the short term. Still, where I saw success most for ulcerative colitis was with diets that included high quality animal proteins.

That said, if you are committed to staying vegan or vegetarian, I have noticed that the diets discussed in this book can be modified for that. My concern would be that it may be difficult to get enough protein, especially in the beginning when there are more limitations on food choices. Since much of the protein in a vegan diet comes from beans, I would consider getting tested for allergies and sensitivities to see if your body will be okay with them, including soy.

If you're a vegetarian and still want to include dairy, I would be tested for that as well. Though, I do personally feel that including dairy in the diet, especially early on, is not optimal. For me, although I am not currently allergic to it, I have noticed that I don't do well with any more than occasional use in small quantities, even if taking digestive enzymes with it. You may not have that issue, but it's important to see how your body reacts.

Another disadvantage of eating vegan or vegetarian is that you would also have to skip the bone broth, which I believe had a huge impact. These are all personal choices. Remember that it's essential to give your body the nutrition it needs to heal and thrive.

As we go through this plan that worked for me, you'll want to know that everything I ingested had to be gluten and dairy free. If I could find the same items free of other potential allergens such as soy, nut and shellfish, that would be preferred as well. However, gluten and dairy were deal breakers. I would not use a product with any dairy or dairy by-products, or gluten. Both could be considered foods that can contribute to inflammation. That even included products such as toothpaste and shampoo, which I often get on my lips as it rinses out.

Now, let's talk about these diets I implemented, one at a time. I'll leave the "how to's" up to other authors and resources that I'll share with you. If you take on any of these diets, you'll want to read up extensively on them. I'll tell you how to do that. Here are the diets and why I chose to implement them.

Specific Carbohydrate Diet

The Specific Carbohydrate Diet (SCD) is a dietary regimen designed to manage certain digestive conditions, particularly inflammatory bowel diseases (IBD) such as Crohn's disease, ulcerative colitis, and irritable bowel syndrome (IBS). The diet was initially developed by Dr. Sidney V. Haas and later popularized by biochemist Elaine Gottschall in her book *Breaking the Vicious Cycle*.

The core principle of the SCD is to eliminate complex carbohydrates that are thought to be challenging to digest. This includes disaccharides and polysaccharides. The theory is that when you eat these types of foods, and they're not digested well or completely, it becomes food for bacteria and parasites. It can also cause damage to your gut lining in addition to your microbiome.

Simply, it seems logical to me to give the digestive system that's already in distress less work to do!

The diet emphasizes the consumption of easily digestible monosaccharides. These are simple sugars that require minimal digestive processing. Theoretically, this can eventually starve out the bad guys taking up residence in your gut.

Processed and refined foods are generally discouraged. The focus is on whole, unprocessed foods to reduce potential irritants and additives. This is common sense!

Foods with gluten are off-limits. This can potentially lower inflammation from the body's reaction to gluten. Many people react to gluten without knowing it. They're not necessarily testing positive for celiac disease, but they have gluten intolerance or sensitivity. Again, this can cause inflammation in the gut. The SCD diet removes that challenge.

Keep in mind that for some people with digestive conditions, gluten may act as an irritant to the intestinal lining, potentially contributing to inflammation and exacerbating symptoms. In individuals with gluten sensitivity, gluten intolerance or celiac disease, the consumption of gluten can trigger an inflammatory response in the small intestine. While the SCD is not specifically designed for those with celiac disease, it shares some principles related to reducing potential irritants.

Gluten is a prominent component of certain grains, particularly wheat, which is widely used in various food products. It's also found in barley and rye. SCD, by restricting certain grains and gluten-containing foods, aligns with its broader goal of eliminating complex carbohydrates.

Studies show that this diet works for ulcerative colitis and Crohn's. The National Library of Medicine site has a number of current published studies on the effectiveness of the Specific Carbohydrate Diet (SCD). You can see it on this link here:

https://www.ncbi.nlm.nih.gov/pmc/?term=%22specific+carbohydrate+diet%22

I strongly suggest buying the book called *Breaking the Viscous Cycle* by Elaine Gottschall. The theory is explained well there, and it's an outstanding resource for getting started with this diet. In fact, I found it essential to have that book on hand.

I'd also suggest joining one or more of the Specific Carbohydrate Diet support groups on Facebook. I found the help invaluable.

Check out a couple websites that have excellent information, including lists of legal and illegal foods and recipes. They are:

- breakingtheviciouscycle.info
- scdrecipe.com

On the Specific Carbohydrate Diet, foods are referred to as either "legal" or "illegal". Ingesting illegal foods can slow down or stall progress. However, in the upcoming chapter where I share the supplements I took to heal from ulcerative colitis, I chose to take an herb called Boswellia although it was illegal. This conflict wasn't a problem for me. I'll discuss this further in the supplement section.

But to be on this diet, I had to stop eating the foods I experienced as the least irritating, including rice, toast, etc. I also chose to stop using marshmallow root tea and the slippery elm capsules which I found to be soothing. They were not allowed. This felt a little counter intuitive. Yet, the science made sense to me, and I wanted to comply with the diet as much as possible.

So, I tried to follow this diet to the letter, to the best of my ability, except for the Boswellia and a couple other things I'll discuss, which I thought of as essential.

There are those who disagree with taking the illegal supplement. However, my theory was that even if I couldn't do the diet perfectly, the degree to which I could follow it could make a very big difference. For me, taking the non-SCD legal supplements I took, especially Boswellia, was the right choice. I kept this type of thing to a minimum though, and only took what I considered high value supplements if they were illegal.

Another element of this diet is that in the beginning, and until you've experienced some healing, you must make sure all your food is cooked. This makes it easier to digest. I even cooked fruit such as cherries and blueberries.

What about juicing?

I've juiced for health for many years, on and off. I've read many books on juicing, and I knew it is commonly used as part of a treatment plan for many illnesses in the holistic community. Some books on ulcerative colitis even recommend it. It's supposed to be easily digestible, so I thought it might be okay despite the rules of this diet. So, I tried it. It was not okay for me until much later, when I was doing much better.

In my research I saw that some people seemed to have success with juicing for ulcerative colitis, especially with cabbage. I did try juicing cabbage at one point fairly early on, after I had experienced some improvement. At that point, I felt that it increased my pain, so I stopped.

It took many months for me to get to the point where I was able to begin eating raw fruits and vegetables again. In the meantime, I found a supplement (Gastrozyme) that had the ingredient in cabbage that was supposed to help with ulcerative colitis. I'll talk about that in the section on supplements I took, but I feel it made a big difference. I was able to get the support without the actual juicing.

Ultimately, I feel this diet had a huge impact on my recovery. I was on it strictly for about 3 years. Some people opt to stay on it forever, but after 3 years I chose to stick with a healthy, balanced organic diet that's gluten and usually dairy free. I also keep the carbs and illegal foods on the lower side.

Although my calprotectin fecal test went up after broadening my diet, it has still stayed well within normal limits. For other health reasons, I periodically go back to this diet along with the Paleo Autoimmune Diet.

One last thought on the SCD diet. For some people, it seems to contain the only dietary changes they need to get well. However, I believe that many people need to go further. SCD doesn't hit all of their root causes.

That's where the Paleo Autoimmune diet comes in. It's my opinion that by combining these diets at least temporarily, it can remove more of the potential root causes. Also, using both of the diets together has the potential to be significantly more anti-inflammatory.

Paleo Autoimmune Diet (AIP)

Since ulcerative colitis can be caused by an autoimmune condition, I chose to use this diet as well. It's also designed to reduce inflammation in the gut, which is exactly what I was looking for. This diet can help the immune system function better.

Paleo Autoimmune removes the foods that cause the highest incidence of allergies and sensitivities. It also removes foods that tend to be more inflammatory such as vegetables considered nightshades (eggplants, peppers, white potatoes, tomatoes, etc.), dairy and gluten.

According to The Paleo Mom, Dr. Sarah Ballantyne's website, it eliminates other foods that are known to contribute towards digestive, health and immune problems including:

- Chemical additives
- Artificial colorings and flavorings
- Legumes (especially soy, peanuts, kidney beans)
- Dairy products
- Trans fats
- High-fructose corn syrup
- Grains including corn
- Pseudograins
- Processed or refined foods
- Refined sugars
- Sugar substitutes (including stevia)
- Refined vegetable oils
- Eggs
- Alcohol
- Coffee
- Nuts
- Seeds

Yes, that's rough.

It's so restrictive that it isn't meant to be permanent in its most restrictive form.

Over time, as you heal, you have the option to reintroduce foods, one at a time, to see how you do. In my opinion, you can also test to see if you have allergies or sensitivities to some of these items on the list. If you don't show a problem with particular foods, it might be okay to add them back in.

Also in my opinion, it would not be wise to reintroduce foods that are known to cause health issues or inflammation, like high-fructose corn syrup, chemical additives, etc. And alcohol kills bacteria, including the good forms. It must be avoided at first, and carefully once healed. Drinking regularly can contribute to losing the ground you took, but if you get to a place where you tolerate it well, drinking alcohol once in a while might be fine for you. You'll be the judge of that.

With dairy, even if not allergic, there may be intolerance, and it may be difficult for some to digest. Lactose intolerance is a problem for many who don't have the natural enzymes (lactase) to digest it properly. Also, it's considered an inflammatory food, so I avoided it completely while healing, and only eat it occasionally now.

Though not specifically on the list, be aware that the Paleo Autoimmune Diet also eliminates gluten. As discussed in the SCD section, removing gluten potentially removes inflammation.

In eliminating gluten, I went all the way. I even changed my toothpaste and mouthwash to brands that were gluten free.

Personally, I went full force on this diet for quite a while. I eliminated anything and everything recommended on the Paleo Autoimmune Diet, and the SCD diet.

Eventually, I had testing done to see if I could add some restricted foods back in. I had blood testing to determine what foods I was allergic to. I also had blood testing to determine what foods I was sensitive to.

As I've mentioned before, food sensitivities are different than allergies. With sensitivities, it can take 2-3 days for reactions to show up, which can make it difficult to identify without testing. This makes it hard to pin down a cause. That's why I feel that blood testing is probably better than experimenting to see how you react.

I continue to test periodically to see if the allergies or sensitivities have changed. Surprisingly, I've found that they do change. Some things I was allergic to for years are now fine for me, and vice-versa. Some things I tested okay for are now on my list of foods to avoid.

Keep in mind that sensitivities can be caused by eating the same things over and over. You may wish to rotate what you eat whenever possible. For me, that just wasn't always practical, so I did develop some sensitivities to foods I frequently ate. However, I still got well eating them, so I'm not sure how far it's necessary to go with avoiding sensitivities. Yet, once I realized I was testing sensitive to foods, I'd eliminate them for a few months. For most foods, this would reverse the sensitivity.

There are several good books on the Paleo Autoimmune Diet, however I found everything I needed online. I'd suggest doing a Google search. There are many sites with lists of foods that are allowed and foods that are not. I'd suggest finding those and printing them out.

A couple sites I've found helpful are:

www.thepaleomom.com

www.autoimmunewellness.com

Low FODMAP Diet

This is designed to help with small intestine bacterial overgrowth or SIBO. I felt it might also help the colon. It eliminates foods with certain sugars that are harder to digest. That sounds a lot like the SCD diet, but they don't completely overlap.

I intended to add this diet to the other two, and I did try to generally stick to those foods that were allowed on the Low FODMAP Diet. But ultimately, I just kept away from foods that were highest on the list to avoid. Garlic and onions were two foods that were allowed on the other diets, but not allowed on this one. In the beginning when my symptoms were severe, I felt that those two things were irritants. It made sense to eliminate them for a while.

However, there were some foods not allowed on the Low FODMAP Diet that I included anyway, and some foods that were allowed that I avoided. Foods such as apples and cherries are not allowed on the Low FODMAP diet but were allowed on the other two diets. Since they didn't seem irritating to me when I cooked them, as per the SCD diet, I included them in my diet.

Since there were many foods that are recommended on the Low FODMAP diet that are not permitted on the other two diets. I gave priority to the SCD and Paleo Autoimmune diets. I used the Low FODMAP diet loosely.

The Maker's Diet

Two very interesting books that I'd recommend reading are *The Maker's Diet* and *Restoring Your Digestive Health*, both by Jordan S. Rubin. Jordan healed himself of Crohn's colitis. These books are packed with helpful information, and I'd highly recommend reading them.

A lot of his suggestions were things I had already implemented in my life, such as eating organic and gluten free.

Many of his recommendations overlapped, at least to some extent, with the diets I was already going to undertake. For example, he recommends limiting grains, and in both of the diets I went on, grains are eliminated altogether.

A couple of big takeaways for me with The Maker's diet were that it's important to eat good quality nutrient dense foods and to supplement with soil-based organisms which I'll discuss coming up. Ultimately, I took away a few additional things from his diet that I implemented, which were in agreement with the other diets I was on. There were also things I was planning to do that The Maker's Diet reinforced. Here are some of these things:

- I included healthy fats in my diet. I got them in the form of coconut oil and olive oil. I also ate avocados and olives. I ate fish at least a couple times a week (it was usually cod or sardines, which I found to be light, easy to digest and I tolerated well).

- The Maker's Diet book reinforced my belief that I didn't need to become vegan to heal.

- I went on a bone broth diet, fasting with only bone broth to rest and support my gut (I added Manuka honey as well). Using bone broth was in alignment with the SCD diet philosophy, and there were studies to back it up.

- I stuck to organic animal-based foods as much as possible, including grass fed/organic meats, organic free-range chickens, and lower mercury wild caught fish such as sardines, salmon, etc.

- I ate blueberries almost daily for the antioxidants and other nutrients, which The Maker's Diet says can help nourish and heal the gut.

- The Maker's Diet included eating organic organ meats such as liver and chicken innards. The liver was something my doctors wanted me on in order to replenish my iron stores. After bleeding for so long, it was important. There are some who are against the eating of organ meats, but I feel it was helpful.

- I took large amounts of soil-based organisms and probiotics (I'll go over these later).

- I cooked with a lot of herbs, especially cinnamon and dill, which have anti-septic properties.

- I took Boswellia root, as I discuss later in this book. It's been one of the keys to healing for me. I had encountered studies early on in my research showing the effectiveness of Boswellia, and The Maker's Diet recommends it.

What did I not do?

In The Maker's Diet book there are some things worth looking at that I wasn't personally able to do, or I chose not to do. You may choose otherwise.

For example:

- It recommended aloe which is known for its ability to soothe the gut. Personally, I'm allergic to it. Also, it's not considered "legal" on the Specific Carbohydrate Diet.

- There are a variety of spices and herbs The Maker's Diet recommends using for various reasons. I chose only the ones I felt were the least irritating to my gut, while providing the most support. I avoided ginger, garlic, etc. These seemed to burn and cause pain. Still, the herbs he includes are worth reading about if you're interested. You may choose differently than I did.

- I chose not to use raw dairy. For me, it appears too risky. There's a chance that raw dairy can introduce infection. Some people I respect seem to believe that it's a part of what can heal the gut, as long as you buy from well-researched and good sources. And others that I respect feel it should be avoided. I chose to skip it, but this is one of those things that may be worth the risk for some. I would suggest you look at the facts and decide for yourself. That said, I healed from ulcerative colitis without it.

- I chose not to eat any dairy at all. It's one of those items on the Paleo Autoimmune Diet that's not allowed. The Maker's Diet includes dairy if it's grass fed, raw, fermented and free of A1 beta casein. For animal sources, it recommends goat, sheep or cow's milk that is free of the A1 beta casein. Again, this is a personal decision. This might be fine for some people. When I experimented with it, it didn't go well for me, so I abstained. That won't be true for everyone.

- Fermented foods tend to be consistently recommended as a part of pretty much every gut restoration plan I've ever seen, including The Maker's Diet. When they're made correctly, they can be loaded with big numbers of probiotics. However, when it came to fermented products such as sauerkraut, Kimchi, and others, for me they seemed to cause esophagus burning and sores in my mouth. I suspect it's because of the high histamine levels. I had to skip all the fermented foods with one exception. I was able to successfully make my own yogurt, which I tolerated well. That is something I started several months into my program, once I was handling food with much less pain. I'll discuss yogurt later in the book.

- I avoided nuts, seeds and nut or seed butter. Though they're allowed on The Maker's Diet, they're not allowed at all in the beginning phase of the Paleo Autoimmune Diet.

Jordan's company, Ancient Nutrition, produces a line of supplements which could be of interest. I did not use them because they were not suitable for my dietary restrictions at the time. Now, I'm seeing what I think are some changes to the ingredients. The relevant products such as collagen and soil-based organisms now appear to be gluten and dairy free, and free of many potential allergens and SCD/AIP off-limits foods. I would personally consider using them now.

Finally, I'd suggest taking a look at an excellent video Jordan produced that you'll find on YouTube called "10 Keys to Conquer Crohn's & Colitis". I found it to be incredibly encouraging, and full of useful information.

What did I eat?

I'm often asked to share what my meals looked like.

First, I'd like to stress the importance of study. As I mentioned before, a big part of my success was diet. To compose the appropriate diet for me, I had to study the SCD book *Breaking the Vicious Cycle*, legal and illegal food lists, etc. I also had to study the Paleo Autoimmune lists of what to avoid, and what to eat.

Back to what I actually ate. My meals were progressive. After fasting for 9-10 days, I followed the Specific Carbohydrate introductory diet minus certain foods that conflicted with the Paleo Autoimmune diet. The introductory diet is meant to be followed when there are severe symptoms such as diarrhea or cramping. In her book, Elaine Gottschall recommends this be followed for up to 5 days if symptoms are severe, and as few as 2 days if they are not. For me, I stayed on this somewhat longer, until I could successfully introduce new foods without severe reactions. That took at least a week to 10 days.

My version of the introductory diet included my home cooked bone broth with the veggies blended, homemade SCD legal gelatin, baked fish, and watered down apple cider. Although beef patties were allowed on both diets, I felt too much increase of pain when eating them, so I skipped them. I was eventually able to add in beef. I don't remember how long it took me, but at least a few months.

As I mentioned, I had to skip SCD allowed foods on the intro diet that conflicted with Paleo Autoimmune, including eggs, yogurt, cottage cheese, and SCD cheesecake. These are all foods that are commonly found to cause allergies, and many people don't have the enzymes needed to digest dairy. While that can be supplemented, I chose not to try. My goal was to remove anything that could have a negative impact on my digestive system.

Honestly, that diet didn't leave a lot of variety. At this point I didn't care. I was looking for relief.

Gradually, as my body allowed, I was able to add in other foods. At first, and for some time, everything had to be cooked. Even fruit. My meals consisted of an organic protein such as chicken or ground turkey, a vegetable such as mushrooms, squash or spinach, and an allowed cooked fruit such as blueberries, applesauce or a ripe banana. I made my own "ices" by cooking down blueberries, adding organic honey, and freezing it in small cups. Eventually, I added my own homemade coconut yogurt to my diet, made with SCD approved probiotic strains.

I used coconut oil, avocado oil and olive oil. When heating food, I tried to stick to the coconut oil which withstands the heat without becoming rancid.

I tried as much as possible to stick with organic. Non-organic food can bring you pesticides, antibiotics, hormones and other toxins. This can change body chemistry. I believe that it's important to remove anything that challenges good health, and to feed the body in a way that encourages life.

During that time, even though allowed on both diets, I also avoided anything acidic or hot such as citrus fruit, garlic, pepper, and onions. Although fruit such as lemon and limes are said to alkalize the body, they're acidic going down, so I avoided them.

Eventually I was able to add back in many foods including citrus, garlic, pepper, onions, beans, nuts, some grains, soy, shellfish, and even occasional dairy. I was also eventually able to eat raw salads, veggies and fruit again, which I was super happy about! It was a gradual process of adding individual items as I felt ready and watching to see how my body reacted.

Also, I continued to avoid foods I tested allergic or sensitive to.

Avoiding Gut irritants - DRUGS

While it's important to avoid food that can irritate the gut, you'll also want to look at your medications. Of course, before you stop anything, check with your doctor who might be able to suggest an alternative.

Some drugs have a direct impact on the gut. For example, NSAID'S such as ibuprofen and aspirin can irritate the digestive system. If possible, refrain from any medications known to irritate or inflame the gut or known to damage the microbiome. I was on a baby aspirin a day when I developed UC. I had to stop it and I've never gone back on it. I had discussed this with my cardiologist, who agreed that I needed to stop the aspirin.

CHAPTER 8: KILLING PARASITES, BACTERIAL AND FUNGAL OVER-GROWTH

As I mentioned before, your doctor should test you for parasites, fungal infection and bacterial infection.

If something comes up positive, you'll probably be put on the appropriate medication. That's a reasonable strategy. There can be downsides to some of these meds, as I've mentioned. For example, antibiotics will kill the good health supporting bacteria in your gut. Still, when you're in the kind of agony that UC can bring on, it might be worth it, if you're able to tolerate the pharmaceuticals. Then afterwards, I would work on correcting any issues caused by the meds, such as a microbiome imbalance.

My doctor tested me for a few of the more common types of bacteria and parasites in my gut. I came up negative.

However, from prior research into this topic, I knew that false negatives are common, especially with parasites. I also knew I was only being tested for a small number of specific bugs.

There are better tests that most mainstream allopathic type doctors don't ordinarily use. Even gastroenterologists. You'd either need a very open-minded doctor who will order a test kit for you, or you'd need a functional/holistic type doctor. You're better off with a doctor who knows how to interpret the results, and who knows how to treat you once the results are in. That means finding a savvy functional or holistic doctor who has studied this test, its interpretation and how to treat based on the results.

As I mentioned before, taking a fecal test such as the one from the Genova lab can give you a wealth of information. This includes what fungus, bacteria and parasites are in your colon, and how much of it is there. It can also tell you if you're missing any good bacteria.

Keep in mind that even though this is considered a good test by many doctors in the holistic/functional community, there can still be false negatives. Especially with parasites which may be in your body but not detected, even in this fecal test.

Through research I have seen that parasites are more common than people think. In the USA we tend to feel we're not exposed. However, parasitic and bacterial infections do not just impact those who have gone to foreign countries. You can get infected anywhere from eating undercooked meats, fish, contaminated water and unwashed foods.

Here's one common example. Have you ever eaten sushi or eaten food prepared on the same surfaces where sushi was made? You may have been exposed to parasites.

There are other ways to be infected such as exposure to blood or feces (who knows where the restaurant chef's hands have been), contaminated dirt or other contaminated surfaces.

My point is that it's possible to pick something up without knowing it, even inside the USA, no matter how careful you are. There are those in the holistic community who believe in doing bi-annual or at least annual parasite cleanses.

Bacterial, fungal and parasitic infections can often be handled naturally, or by using drugs. Some, even within the holistic community, feel the drugs are necessary when it comes to parasites. Others treat only using natural alternatives. There are many good quality antiparasitic products you'll find at the health food store or online.

Personally, I tended to have allergies to a couple of the common ingredients in natural parasite cleanse products. I was also hesitant to use a lot of herbals since my colon was in such distress. So, in the beginning of treating myself, I did not take anything specifically for parasites. Instead, I took on a diet (SCD) that could starve parasites and bad bacteria. I'll talk more about the diet in a minute.

Years later I found some products that were tolerable and effective, though I haven't tried them while having active ulcerative colitis symptoms. They are from the company called Cellcore. I've used Para 1 and Para 2 with success. Personally, had I known about these, I would have taken them early on.

The antiparasitic formulas are supposed to be taken with binder formulas that include carbon. They are designed to mop up any toxins the parasites give off when they die. However, I have found that these binder products irritated my gut. Even to this day I feel discomfort if I take binders. So, I just take Cellcore Para 1 and Para 2. In chapter 14, I mention some more gentle, natural binders.

At the start of my self-treatment, I took some gentle natural antibacterials for a few weeks. I had done well with them in the past and found them gentle on the gut. Over the years I've found that these products have been helpful and effective at getting rid of many bacterial infections I had experienced.

I will say that I believe there are times when an antibiotic is necessary despite the side effects and the fact that they usually kill the good flora in your gut. Since I have not reacted well to pharmaceutical antibiotics in the past, I started out researching and using the natural options.

There were four strategies that I used to deal with this issue:

1. Herbs
2. Colloidal silver

3. Diet
4. Replenishing microbiome balance

I'll go over what I took, and I'll add a section to the book with the brands I took along with dosages. All the products I use are researched to fit into the boundaries of the diets I'll talk about coming up. As with the Boswellia, if the substance itself didn't fit in, at least the other ingredients in the supplements did.

Herbs and Colloidal Silver

As I've mentioned, some herbs and colloidal silver are known to have antibacterial, antiparasitic, antiviral and antifungal properties.

Grapefruit seed extract also has the ability to break down biofilm colonies. Biofilms are the coming together of microorganisms such as bacteria that adhere to each other and to surfaces, creating a slimy protective matrix. Biofilm formation allows bacteria to resist the host immune system, antibiotic treatments, and other environmental stresses.

Grapefruit seed extract is believed by some to have properties that can interfere with the formation and integrity of bacterial biofilms. I took this along with other herbs and silver.

For me and for many others, these natural herbs and substances tend to have less side effects than pharmaceuticals. In my experience, they may not be as strong as the pharmaceutical drugs, but they have worked for me.

I wanted to kill any bad bacteria that I could up front, without making the gut inflammation worse. In the past I'd take the name of a specific type of bacteria I had been diagnosed with such as in a urine test, and search for studies that verify the effectiveness of specific herbs on that bacterium. You'd be surprised at how many studies have been done, showing the effectiveness of herbs.

I've done this with success many times.

Since I didn't have the name of a specific bacterial infection, my theory was that by using a variety of natural herbs, I could hopefully kill whatever was in there that shouldn't be. My intention was to use as many things as I could tolerate to send out a wide spread of "bullets", so to speak.

Even if it didn't knock out everything that shouldn't be there, at least I could reduce the load so my body would have less work to do. The idea was to regain balance.

For about 3-4 weeks I took the following:

- Goldenseal root
- Olive leaf extract
- Berberine
- Grapefruit seed extract
- Colloidal silver

These are my favorite herbs and supplements for this purpose. I find them to be easy on the gut, and well tolerated.

There are others that might be helpful. Since that time, an herb that I learned about was cryptolepis tincture. I've found it also to be gentle on the gut and effective.

I have found a couple other natural antibacterials to be harsh on the gut. I have seen these recommended for ulcerative colitis, but in my opinion that would be counterproductive. Though they might be effective at killing bacteria and even some parasites, I felt that I couldn't afford to increase the inflammation in my colon. I chose to avoid them. Those herbals include oregano oil and black seed oil. Personally, I would only use these once healed, and then sparingly, if other things are not working.

Colloidal silver has been in my medicine chest for over 30 years. I've even owned a silver generator so that I could make my own. If you look up colloidal silver on the internet, you'll see articles galore that talk about a condition called argyria. This is where the skin turns grayish-bluish. As I said, I've been taking it for decades as needed, and have not developed this condition, and I don't know of anyone who has. Taking good quality silver as needed has worked fine for me.

I have found silver to be helpful with infections. I can't say that it's strong enough to get by with alone, usually. But I've found it to be a helpful part of my arsenal.

Another way to deal with parasites and bacteria is through diet. If you check out the diets I mentioned previously, you'll see that they can help with this issue. The Specific Carbohydrate Diet is specially designed for this.

Chapter 8: Killing Parasites, Bacterial and Fungal Overgrowth

CHAPTER 9: SUPPLEMENTS TO REDUCE COLON INFLAMMATION AND/OR TO HEAL THE GUT

I'm going to share what supplements I chose to take. For most of them, I took them for a couple years. However, the one supplement that I continue to take to this day is at the top of my list, Boswellia Serrata.

Since I tend to be sensitive, whenever I start a new supplement, I start low and slow. It's important to make sure my body tolerates the new supplement well. Often, if it's in capsule form, I'll open it and remove much of the ingredients, close it, and then take what's left. If it's a tablet, as long as it doesn't have a special coating, I'll break off a piece and take it. Then, if all goes well, I'll gradually raise my dose, making sure my body is accepting the supplement at the new dosage. Unless there's urgency, I'll usually introduce one supplement at a time, over several days.

Here are the supplements:

Boswellia Serrata

In my research, I was looking for something natural that would be the equivalent of the prescription drug Mesalamine, that my doctor had prescribed. Thankfully I found studies that showed Boswellia serrata was a winner.

Boswellia is made from the bark of the Boswellia tree, but it's also known as frankincense. Yes, the famous frankincense that was part of the gifts that the Three Wise Men brought to Jesus in the manger. It definitely does have healing ability.

In the book called Integrative Medicine (Fourth Edition), the following is said:

> "Boswellia *is believed to act via inhibition of 5-lipoxygenase, thereby decreasing leukotriene biosynthesis and resulting in diminished proinflammatory cytokine release. A small trial of active UC patients found that* Boswellia *350 mg three times a day was as effective as sulfasalazine 1000 mg three times a day in decreasing symptoms and laboratory indicators. A second similar study of 30 active UC patients again found* Boswellia *to be as effective as sulfasalazine, with remission rates of 82% and 75%, respectively.* Boswellia *has also been tested in Crohn patients for initiating and maintaining remission. Gerhardt et al. performed a randomized, double-blinded study of 102 patients comparing H15, a proprietary* Boswellia serrata *extract, to mesalazine and found a similar decrease in*

CDAI in both groups, showing that Boswellia *is noninferior to mesalamine for treatment of CD. Holtmeier et al. evaluated* Boswellia *versus placebo for maintenance of remission in CD and found no significant difference, but did confirm excellent tolerability and minimal adverse effects."*

CD is Crohn's Disease, and CDAI is the Crohn's Disease Activity Index. Mesalazine is the same drug as mesalamine. Sulfasalazine is similar to mesalamine, except it has sulfa in it which can cause some people side effects.

So, according to this, for Crohn's and ulcerative colitis, Boswellia can be just as effective as the drugs mesalamine and sulfasalazine. With ulcerative colitis, Boswellia had a higher remission rate than the drug sulfasalazine.

For me, it's been highly effective with no side effects. It's the one supplement I've continued to take long after the symptoms and inflammation have gone.

The only issue with Boswellia is that it is not permitted on the Specific Carbohydrate Diet, and I wasn't able to locate anything else that had the same results as Boswellia. When I saw this, I realized I had a decision to make. Either I'd need to take the drug mesalamine, or I'd need to take the Boswellia even though it's considered "illegal" on the SCD diet. For me, that was an easy decision. Though Boswellia would not assist with the aims of the SCD diet, it has far less side effects than the mesalamine. It was also radically less expensive. I took the

Boswellia and found that everything worked together effectively. That's despite it being illegal.

Keep in mind that there are those who would disagree with my choice. In fact, I was a member of one particularly helpful Facebook support group for the SCD diet. I was not permitted to mention the Boswellia, even though it was so effective for me. The admins would delete any post where I said I was taking it. They seemed to believe that nothing less than maintaining SCD perfectly would be okay. It was their group, so I had to respect their rules, but it wasn't my experience. I felt sad that I couldn't share this with some very desperate people who could have benefited.

One last thing about Boswellia. In the essential oil form called frankincense, it's supposed to be more powerful than using it as Boswellia. I have not tried this, but plan to add it in at some point, just to see if I experience a difference. It may be worth considering.

Collagen Powder

I didn't use this at first, but eventually, after a couple years, I got tired of making the bone broth so frequently. I wanted to continue feeding my colon good building and healing materials, although I felt well at this point.

I realized that I could get at least some of the mucosal healing ingredients found in the soup by using collagen powder.

I've found that it makes a difference to the gut, and as a bonus, it helps with muscles, bones, connective tissues and hair.

I don't think I'd replace the bone broth with this while healing, but if I could go back in time, I would have added this to my plan. Now, I put a scoop in my coffee whenever I have a cup.

There are many good brands of collagen powder on the market, and I shift based on price. I look for hydrolyzed and agglomerated bovine collagen powder, preferably pasture raised, organic. As with everything, make sure it's gluten free. It should have type I and III collagen.

Digestive Enzymes

This was an important part of the process. I took digestive enzymes whenever I ate.

I did not take an enzyme product that included the acids (hydrochloric acid or bile acids), as I felt that it wasn't going to work out well with all the ulcers I had.

The goal was to assist my digestive process so my body didn't have to deal with undigested food which can create problems leading to inflammation and leaky gut. And of course, it's essential for healing to have the right nutrition from food. If there's ulcerative colitis going on, I believe that you can assume you're not digesting your food optimally.

I found a product that I felt fit in with the diets and restrictions I had, while providing helpful levels of enzymes, etc. That was Digest Gold by Enzymedica. I took 1-3 capsules each time I ate, depending on the quantity of food. If I ate a small non-fatty meal I would use one Digest Gold. If I ate more, I would take more capsules. If the meal was fatty, I'd also add Enzymedica's Lypo Gold product.

Gastrazyme

Juicing cabbage is known to have healing properties for the gut lining; however, I could not get it down without a lot of pain. Additionally, it's a lot of work to juice! Not to mention that I found the taste repulsive.

Enter Gastrazyme made by Biotics Research. This supplement has the vitamin U complex found in cabbage juice. Plus, it has other supplements that support healing of the gut lining. You get all the benefits with none of the difficulties. Honestly, I don't know why, but I found this supplement reduced pain quickly. Next to Boswellia, this seemed to bring the quickest results.

L-Glutamine

The many ways that L-glutamine can help heal the gut had me including this. It potentially helps heal leaky gut, reduces inflammation, and more. There are some contradictory studies though, with some showing that it works to help heal the gut, and some showing no improvement. I felt that the pro glutamine studies were compelling enough to make it worth a try. Plus, I had a couple of functional doctors recommend it.

IMPORTANT: Please note that for anyone dealing with cancer, glutamine may be a supplement to avoid. It may feed cancer.

Zinc-L-Carnosine

This is healing to ulcers. Zinc-L-Carnosine has been studied quite a bit for its potential therapeutic effects on various gastrointestinal conditions, including ulcers. Just do a Google search and you'll see many studies with positive outcomes. There are so many ways in which this compound can help.

Zinc is an essential mineral that plays a crucial role in wound healing and tissue repair. When combined with L-carnosine, it forms a complex that has been shown to enhance the healing of gastric mucosa, the protective lining of the stomach.

L-carnosine has anti-inflammatory properties, and inflammation is a significant factor in the development and exacerbation of ulcers. By reducing inflammation, Zinc-L-Carnosine may contribute to the healing process.

Studies suggest that Zinc-L-Carnosine has gastroprotective effects, helping to protect the stomach lining from damage caused by factors such as excess gastric acid and certain medications.

Mucins are proteins that form a protective layer over the stomach lining. Zinc-L-Carnosine is thought to stimulate the production of mucins, enhancing the protective barrier and promoting ulcer healing.

Helicobacter pylori is a bacterium associated with the development of peptic ulcers. Some studies suggest that Zinc-L-Carnosine may help inhibit the growth of H. pylori, potentially aiding in the treatment of ulcers associated with this bacterium.

Zinc-L-Carnosine may modulate the production of pro-inflammatory cytokines, substances that play a role in the inflammatory response. By regulating these cytokines, the compound may contribute to a more balanced and controlled inflammatory environment in the stomach.

So, zinc-L-carnosine is a winner when it comes to ulcerative colitis. I took 20 mg daily of a product by Doctor's Best called PepZin GI.

CHAPTER 10: REPLENISHING THE GUT FLORA

Navigating the complex terrain of ulcerative colitis often requires a multifaceted approach, and one pivotal player in this healing journey is the intricate ecosystem of your gut. In this chapter, we'll delve into the art of replenishing good bacteria, exploring the role of probiotics, with a special focus on soil-based organisms and their synergy with other probiotic strains.

Understanding the Gut Microbiome

Your gut is home to trillions of microorganisms, collectively known as the gut microbiome. Among them, bacteria play a crucial role in maintaining a delicate balance that influences your overall health, including the well-being of your digestive system.

When our guts are functioning properly, the microscopic bacterial inhabitants inside you are balanced. The gut thrives on diversity with a robust and diverse microbial community. While there might be some bad players in there, in a healthy gut they're kept in check by the good guys. If the good guys get knocked off and the bad guys gain ground, it can cause all kinds of health problems, including ulcerative colitis.

The microbiome makes up a large part of your immune system. A well-balanced gut microbiome, supported by a variety of probiotic strains, can contribute to a balanced immune response, crucial in managing conditions including ulcerative colitis.

Many things can cause an imbalance, killing off the good guys or causing too many bad guys to flourish. For example, drugs such as antibiotics cause the death of both good and bad bacteria, which could allow funguses to thrive.

Too much sugar in your diet can cause an imbalance. Combine a diet with a lot of sugar with a round of antibiotics and you've got a breeding ground for an overgrowth of fungus and bad bacteria that whichever antibiotic you took didn't kill. As discussed above, parasites that have taken up residence can also flourish when there's a flora imbalance.

How did I Improve gut flora?

In a prior chapter I talked about killing off the bad bacteria, excess fungus and parasites in the gut. That's all important, but so is focusing on replenishing the good bacteria.

First, as I mentioned in prior sections, diet is a huge part of what can influence that. The right diet can starve out the bad stuff while feeding the good stuff. It can help create an atmosphere that helps, supports and nurtures the good bacteria.

It's also important to take some good bacteria orally. Most people know that there are probiotics in food such as yogurt. However, the products you see in the grocery store for the most part either have dead organisms, a small number of organisms, or organisms that are not necessarily going to help with healing the gut. That's why it's important to supplement with the right, high potency probiotics.

Different strains of probiotics seem to impact the body in different ways. There were a couple of strains that I found have shown to help heal ulcerative colitis, and/or Crohn's.

The Probiotics I Took

I was impressed by the impact that something called soil-based organisms had on Jordan Rubin's ulcerative colitis condition, as described in his books I mentioned previously. According to him they played a huge role in turning around his health. I decided to take a product that included soil-based organisms (Bacillus Subtilis HU58) along with other strains of bacteria that are known for supporting the gut.

The product is made by Silver Fern and called Ultimate Probiotic. I worked up to 6 capsules a day, and for a short time, I took even more (as many as 12 capsules a day). This product didn't appear to have any "illegal" ingredients according to the SCD diet, although that diet's creator was not recommending these particular probiotic strains. Still, I chose to use this anyway.

One of the strains this product contains is called bacillus coagulans. Known for its resilience, Bacillus coagulans is believed to survive the harsh environment of the stomach and reach the intestines intact, contributing to gut health.

There is also something in this product called saccharomyces boulardii or S. boulardii. This is a beneficial yeast that is associated with reducing inflammation and supporting the intestinal barrier.

This product seemed to make a difference for me.

Another probiotic strain I chose to use is Lactobacillus plantarum 299v. Studies on this strain showed significant support for ulcerative colitis. According to one study, it did the following for mice:

> *"Lactobacillus plantarum 299v prevented onset of disease and reduced established colitis."*

I used the product from Jarrow Formulas called Ideal Bowel Support and took a capsule a day for more than a year. After that, I still took it on and off. It's dairy and gluten free.

What about prebiotics? Prebiotics are foods that the probiotics feed on. The SCD diet recommends not to take prebiotics as they believe this could feed the bad stuff. There are some natural foods that are on the legal SCD list that do feed the probiotics anyway, such as onions and asparagus. Though I didn't eat onions until I was feeling much better, I did eat asparagus fairly early on. I followed the recommendation of the SCD diet and did not supplement with prebiotics.

The SCD diet also recommends avoiding the Bifidobacteria strains of probiotics. They believe it can contribute to the overgrowth of bad bacteria in the gut. Upon researching, I saw that this was controversial. Some studies find that it can benefit those with irritable bowel disease. Regardless, I did avoid it for the first couple years. I am currently on a product which includes it, and I'm doing fine.

Homemade Yogurt

As mentioned before, I did not do well with fermented foods in the beginning, and most of them (if not all) are too challenging to digest with active ulcerative colitis. However, I did seem to tolerate small amounts of homemade yogurt.

After several months on my program, and after the bleeding stopped and the symptoms calmed down, I felt I could take this on and give it a try. Although cooking is challenging for me physically, I felt that the more probiotics I could get in, the better.

I decided to make my own non-dairy version of the Specific Carbohydrate Diet yogurt. Remember, the Paleo Autoimmune Diet specifically calls for no dairy. However, on the SCD diet dairy based yogurt is included as a more advanced food meant to be started after significant healing and progress has been made. I chose to stay off dairy.

Although there are non-dairy yogurts galore in the health food store, none of them complied with the various SCD diet limitations. They also contained strains of probiotics that were not necessarily best or enough for me. These are all reasons why I needed to make my own yogurt.

I purchased a simple yogurt maker on Amazon, which allowed me to make 8 cups of yogurt at a time.

Non-Dairy Milk: I used Native Forest Simple Organic Unsweetened Coconut Milk cans as a base. It has to be the "simple" version which leaves out the Guar, which is illegal on the SCD food list. I got this on Amazon, buying a case at a time.

In dairy based milk, the probiotics feed on the lactose in the milk. If you're using non-dairy milk, it's going to be necessary to add honey for the probiotics to feed on, and gelatin for texture. More on that is coming up.

Starter: When making yogurt, you need a starter. This is the probiotic that will grow in your yogurt as you allow it to cook and ferment. I used an SCD approved brand from GI ProHealth called GI ProStart. It contains L. Bulgaricus, S. Thermophilus and L. Casei, which can turn milk or non-dairy milk into yogurt. It's dairy and gluten free. You can find the yogurt starter on this site:

https://giprohealth.com/products/gi-prostart-yogurt-starter

Sweetener & Flavor: As I mentioned, non-dairy yogurt must have something to feed the good bacteria. So, honey was a necessary ingredient. I sweetened the yogurt with organic unfiltered honey (make sure it's gluten free) and added some fruit such as blueberries or cherries.

Gelatin: The non-dairy recipe calls for gelatin, which in itself is healing to the gut. According to WebMD the proteins in gelatin can help support the intestinal wall, including building the protective mucus lining in your intestines. It can help protect the lining of the intestines.

Cooking Directions: To find cooking directions for making SCD compliant non-dairy yogurt, check out this site and page here:

https://www.nimbal.org/education/preparing-scd-food/making-scd-yogurt

One thing of note. The recipe on that page has you making your own coconut milk. As mentioned, I didn't do that. However, if you're ambitious and like to cook, go for it. Fresh is always better.

Here's another helpful resource.

There are good directions for cooking a dairy based SCD compliant yogurt on the following site. Though I don't consider using dairy while healing a good idea, these cooking directions explain parts of the process well. While you're there, check out the rest of the site. It's an extremely helpful site with plenty of tips for following the SCD diet and for making your yogurt.

The site and page are here:

https://breakingtheviciouscycle.info/how-to-make-scd-yogurt

Adding Yogurt to Your Diet: After making the yogurt for the first time, I was pleased to find that it was actually pretty good! And it was nice to be able to eat something new.

I started out eating a spoon full and worked my way up to a cup 3-7 times a week. Since it had fat in it, I took digestive enzymes with it – both Digest Gold and Lypo Gold.

Probiotic I'm Currently Taking

At this time, I'm using a probiotic product by Dr. Ruscio, DNM DC. He is someone who's done a great deal of research on healing the gut. I've found that he's very research-based and has a focus on treating gut dysfunction.

The product is called Triple Therapy Probiotic Powder Sticks. It comes in the form of single-dose packets with powder. These probiotic packets each contain three categories of helpful probiotics. It has the soil-based organisms, lactobacillus strains, and saccharomyces boulardii in it. It also does have some bifidobacterium that are not legal on the SCD diet, but I'm not convinced that it's a bad thing. As I mentioned, some studies show it can help.

I moved over to this product because I like the convenience of having all three types of probiotics in one packet. I also feel that Dr. Ruscio has done his research into the impact of certain strains of probiotics on ulcerative colitis. Also, varying strains seems like logic to me when rebuilding the gut flora.

On the other hand, by having the various probiotics separate initially, I was able to build up slowly without encountering any side effects. I was able to gauge the impact of each product. There's something to be said for starting slow and low, and building up as the body allows.

CHAPTER 11: WATER QUALITY

Something that I've always considered essential to health is water quality. The chemicals present in tap water can have various effects on the human microbiome, the community of trillions of microbes that inhabit the gastrointestinal tract and other mucosal surfaces.

While tap water is treated to meet safety standards and is generally considered safe for consumption, the presence of certain chemicals may have unintended consequences on the microbiome (and the rest of the body).

For example, chlorine and chloramine are commonly used disinfectants in water treatment plants to eliminate harmful bacteria and pathogens. However, they can also affect beneficial bacteria in the microbiome of those drinking the water.

These chemicals may disrupt the balance of gut bacteria, potentially leading to alterations in the diversity and composition of the microbiome.

Also, some tap water may contain trace amounts of heavy metals like lead, copper, and cadmium, which can have antimicrobial properties.

Residues of pharmaceuticals, including antibiotics, may be present in trace amounts in tap water. Prolonged exposure to low levels of antibiotics may contribute to the development of antibiotic-resistant strains of bacteria in the gut.

Fluoride is often added to tap water to prevent dental cavities. While the primary purpose is dental health, excessive fluoride exposure may have unintended effects on gut bacteria. Studies have suggested that fluoride can cause other serious illnesses as well (I use non-fluoride toothpaste to protect the flora in my mouth and gut).

To mitigate potential negative effects of tap water, consider using water filters designed to remove specific contaminants.

We have always used water filters in our home. The challenge is that the pH level of filtered water can be acidic.

The pH level of drinking water refers to its acidity or alkalinity, with a pH scale ranging from 0 to 14. A pH of 7 is considered neutral, while values below 7 indicate acidity, and values above 7 indicate alkalinity. The pH level of drinking water can impact its taste, corrosiveness, and potential health effects.

Many water filtering devices create water that is acidic because they remove all the bad stuff, but also the good minerals that make water neutral or alkaline. Water that has been through reverse osmosis or that is distilled tends to be acidic.

It's my belief that water that's acidic can be irritating to ulcerative colitis.

Spring water usually has an alkaline pH, and I chose to drink spring water or water from a filter we already had that creates neutral or alkaline levels in the water it outputs. That filter is called the Jupiter Melody Water Ionizer sold by Alka-Viva.

Our unit is quite old and ultimately, we were not convinced the Jupiter Melody model was purifying as completely as we wished. There are newer versions of this water filter that offer more efficient filtration. They also create molecular hydrogen in the water, which is an antioxidant.

Hydrogen water is getting a lot of attention lately for its healing ability. Apparently, studies indicate that hydrogen water can help with gut healing. It's known for bringing down inflammation in the body, including in the gut.

If money was not an issue, this is what I'd do:

I'd use a reverse osmosis filter system as a pre-filter to remove impurities as fully as possible. I'd then have the water output by that system go through an AlkaViva ionizer/hydrogen maker. Reverse osmosis is known to be an effective filtration system. By combining the two systems, the resulting water would be highly filtered, alkaline, with molecular hydrogen in the water.

The people at AlkaViva can help you figure out how to accomplish this. We're not associated with them, other than as a client.

We have not been ready to invest in a new water system because of the expense. So, we have rigged up a less expensive process. We are currently taking the water that comes out of the Jupiter Melody and putting it through a Burkey water filter to get it more pure.

Burkey makes filters that are highly effective according to their published test results, and they're very reasonably priced. Their water filters are supposed to create an alkaline pH. We purchased their pre-filter that removes fluoride and arsenic from the water to get the best possible filtration they provide.

Using both water filter devices together, we've found that our water is coming out alkaline. We believe it's being adequately filtered, and it tastes good. We may be losing some of the ionization of the water by adding a second filter, but we're not sure. Still, we're comfortable with the level of filtration and the pH.

I'm sure there are other good water filtration solutions out there as well that would be efficient. If I were considering one, I'd look for the highest purity, with a water output that's at least a neutral pH. A Google search will bring up some water filters that use reverse osmosis but create alkaline or neutral pH water.

Personally, I decided not to have the water come out highly alkaline. Our digestive systems need some acid for digestion, and I feel it's important not to overdo the alkalinity. I've chosen to stick to a neutral or slightly alkaline pH with my water.

In addition to using the system we put together, I recently purchased some inexpensive hydrogen water units on Amazon.com for home use. They take your water and infuse hydrogen into it. I'm just beginning to try out hydrogen infused water. It's too early to tell if it will make a difference to my health, but I figure it's added support, and might assist with keeping my gut healthy.

CHAPTER 12: OTHER SUPPLEMENTS THAT MIGHT BE HELPFUL

There are a couple other things that I was already taking which could be considered as supportive for gut healing. I'll talk about those, as well as iron, which I needed because of the bleeding I experienced.

Methyl B12 and Methyl Folate

Many people are unaware that there's a genetic mutation test that can identify a problem which is easily treatable and can cause serious repercussions if not treated.

People with MTHFR variants may experience challenges in processing folate and B12 efficiently. Folate and B12 are essential vitamins that undergo a conversion process to their methylated forms for proper utilization by the body. MTHFR gene variations can impact this conversion, leading to potential difficulties in effectively utilizing these vitamins.

Inadequate levels of B12 or folate in the body may give rise to various health issues. These vitamins play crucial roles in processes such as DNA synthesis, red blood cell formation, and nervous system function. When the conversion process is hindered by MTHFR variants, it can contribute to health challenges.

The impact of MTHFR variants varies among individuals, and not everyone with these variations will experience the same level of difficulty in processing B12 and folate. I've found that addressing these challenges often involves personalized approaches, such as targeted supplementation and lifestyle adjustments.

An excellent source of information on this subject is a site by Dr. Ben Lynch, here:

https://mthfr.net/

The impact of MTHFR variants on folate and B12 metabolism can have implications for those with ulcerative colitis. In the context of UC, where inflammation and nutritional challenges are common, proper folate and B12 utilization becomes particularly crucial.

The compromised conversion process associated with MTHFR variants may exacerbate nutrient deficiencies, potentially contributing to symptoms and complicating the management of UC.

Insufficient levels of these vitamins can affect the integrity of the gastrointestinal lining, immune function, and overall well-being. So, those with UC and MTHFR variants may benefit from close monitoring of their nutritional status, and personalized supplementation strategies. Personally, I have blood tests checking my B12 status regularly through an anti-aging/functional doctor.

On Dr. Lynch's site, there are some great articles on how to supplement for your specific genetic variants. I also use some of his products as long as they're gluten and dairy free. Not all of them are, so it's important to check.

Personally, I have this kind of genetic variant. When I developed UC, I was already on the methylated forms of b12 and folate, as well as a b-complex supplement. How much to take is so different for each person, that I won't share dosages. Instead, I'd recommend talking with a knowledgeable doctor, and getting tested for this genetic issue.

If your test comes back as positive for a mutation, especially if it's homozygous (from both parents), I'd suggest reading books on the subject and joining Facebook forums to learn more about what works and what doesn't. It's a complex subject and one that has entire books dedicated to it.

Doctors can prescribe a blood or saliva test to determine your genetic status. My doctor did a blood test on me, and I also went through the site called www.23andme.com for genetic testing. Your doctor can also test your b12 and folate status through blood.

Iron

If you've been bleeding, you may be low on iron. Your doctor may have told you to take iron supplements. Many iron supplements can be hard on the stomach. I was unable to handle iron supplements for quite some time.

Instead, early in my program I ate liver just about every other day. This slowly helped but didn't get me to normal levels.

Eventually, when my gut was a lot better, I was able to use a liquid iron product which I diluted. I tolerated it much better than several other products I had tried. It was made by Gaia Herbs and called Plant Force Liquid Iron. How much you'd take would depend on your deficiency level.

I would suggest being closely monitored when taking iron, as this is a vitamin that you can have too much of. Iron toxicity is something to avoid.

Magnesium

I discovered that it was very important to not allow myself to get constipated. It seemed to stall and reverse progress with gut healing. What works great for me is to take magnesium.

It keeps my bowels moving properly, given the right dose, and it's also good for many other conditions.

To counter constipation, there are times where I've taken 600-700 mg twice a day to keep my bowels moving at least once or twice a day. The dose has been trial and error, because too much can cause diarrhea or unformed bowel movements. As always, when I start a supplement, I choose to start slow and low. 100-200 mg a day was the starting point for me.

Some forms of magnesium are more easily absorbed by the body such as magnesium glycinate, so you may need a higher dose to impact the bowels. Other forms are not as well absorbed and might work to get the bowels moving with less milligrams, such as with magnesium oxide or magnesium citrate.

I have had very good results with a mixture of magnesium forms in a product called Target-Mins Magnesium Caps with silica by Country Life.

Dealing with Glyphosate with Citrus Pectin, Fulvic Acid & Humic Acid, Milk Thistle

Glyphosate is a chemical found in weed killer and it's commonly used. It's also found in many common foods since it's used in farming. Glyphosate can increase the likelihood and severity of ulcerative colitis, even at levels deemed safe by the EPA. It's known to disrupt the gut microbiota.

To remove it from the body, one of the things that can work according to Dr. Josh Axe is Citrus pectin. It's a soluble fiber known to detoxify heavy metals and clear cholesterol through its binding powers. I've used a product called Pectasol which has studies behind it and have found it to be very gentle on my gut.

One of my doctors highly recommends ION Gut Support which has fulvic acid and humic acid. These are known to bind to glyphosate in the GI tract to help transport it out. This supplement is also known to strengthen the lining of the gut, so I consider it a good idea as a part of a healing protocol. Although I didn't take it while healing initially, I'm currently using it to support my gut. Here's where you'll find it:

https://intelligenceofnature.com/products/gut-health-supplement

Supporting the liver is also a way to help the body deal with glyphosate. My favorite liver support herb is milk thistle. I always take it whenever I take Tylenol to protect my liver. I also take it regularly to heal and protect the liver. I've found it to be very effective over the years.

Chapter 12: Other Supplements that Might Be Helpful

CHAPTER 13: SUPPLEMENTS & DRUGS I DIDN'T USE, WHICH MIGHT BE HELPFUL

There are a couple of supplements and drugs that I did not choose to take or couldn't take due to allergies. They might be worth considering. Though this book is about healing naturally, sometimes a drug can be helpful. The drugs I'll mention are light on the side effects compared with some of the ulcerative colitis drugs, so they might be worth considering.

Histamine blockers

If you suspect a histamine issue, (mast cell activation syndrome or histamine intolerance), it might be worth considering taking a histamine-1 and histamine-2 blocker. Claritin blocks histamine-1 (H1) and Pepcid blocks histamine-2 (H2). As mentioned in this book, bone broth as well as fermented foods can contain histamine. These over-the-counter meds could be taken to counter histamine. Naturally, they're not without possible side effects, so it's important to consider whether the benefits would make it worthwhile.

A more natural solution that might be helpful is quercetin, though I'm not sure it compares to the medicines mentioned above when it comes to effectiveness. Other natural antihistamine options you could add include vitamin C, stinging nettle, butterbur and bromelain. Of course, some of these might be acidic, such as the vitamin C, so use carefully. I found that even the buffered vitamin C was irritating to my gut.

Low Dose Naltrexone (LDN)

I'm not a person that tends to use medications. In fact, I tend to do the opposite whenever possible. This is one of the few drugs that I think is fantastic. I was allergic to this drug, or I would have been on it.

While naltrexone is an anti-opiate used to treat opiate addiction and alcohol dependence, used in very small doses, it's an immune modulator. This means it can help work against autoimmunity, one of the possible root causes of ulcerative colitis. It does this without suppressing the immune system as some of the ulcerative colitis medications do. Rather it helps to balance the immune system.

I've followed several LDN focused forums, and I've seen story after story about the way LDN changed people's health.

As I mentioned, LDN is believed to have immunomodulatory effects, meaning it may help regulate the immune system. In autoimmune conditions like ulcerative colitis, where the immune system attacks the digestive tract, modulating immune responses could potentially reduce inflammation.

Also, LDN is thought to stimulate the release of endorphins, the body's natural painkillers. Endorphins may contribute to overall well-being and potentially help alleviate symptoms associated with ulcerative colitis.

There is some evidence suggesting that LDN might improve gut barrier function, helping to maintain the integrity of the intestinal lining. Some individuals with ulcerative colitis report improvements in symptoms such as abdominal pain, diarrhea, and fatigue with the use of LDN.

I'd been trying to get on this drug for years because I've seen so much success reported with it for illnesses such as MS, cancer and Lyme disease. And as far as side effects are concerned, there are very few. It seems to be amazing. Unfortunately, I have remained allergic to it.

In some small studies, it's shown effective for ulcerative colitis and Crohn's. In my opinion, this is worth trying. Especially if you suspect that you have an autoimmune issue which could be the root cause of ulcerative colitis.

Unfortunately, Low Dose Naltrexone is an off-label use of Naltrexone. It may not be covered by insurance. You will need a prescription, but most mainstream doctors don't know about it, and won't prescribe it. This would require an alternative doctor who has looked into it, such as a functional or anti-aging doctor.

Many people purchase their LDN through Skip's Pharmacy in Deerfield Beach, Florida. We've found them to be knowledgeable and helpful there.

Sodium Butyrate

Although I didn't include this, it has potential to assist in healing ulcerative colitis. Sodium butyrate has anti-inflammatory properties, and it supports intestinal barrier function which may help strengthen the epithelial lining of the colon. It's a preferred energy source for the cells lining the colon (colonocytes). It can also play a role in regulating the immune response in the gut.

It's most effective taken rectally. Rectal forms of sodium butyrate, such as suppositories or enemas, are designed to deliver the supplement directly to the colon. This can be particularly beneficial when the inflammation in ulcerative colitis is localized to the lower part of the colon (rectum or sigmoid colon). Rectal administration allows for targeted delivery of the supplement to the affected area. It can also be taken orally, but it may not work as effectively.

Tumeric (curcumin)

Although I tried turmeric capsules, I did not feel that it was making a difference for me. However, this herb is known for its anti-inflammatory and antioxidant properties. The more I learn about it, the more I feel that I may not have given it enough time to work.

I've seen it frequently recommended for gut healing. Even though I got well without using it long-term, it has potential because of all the known benefits. It's something to be considered.

CHAPTER 14: IF YOU'VE HAD MOLD EXPOSURE

Mold exposure can wreak havoc on your body, and it is a potential root cause of ulcerative colitis.

If you test positive on a mycotoxin test (see the test section of the book), detoxing the mycotoxins will be important for your health. The first step will be to find the source of the exposure and fix it. Often, this will require using a professional mold remediation company. You can make things worse if you try to do it yourself.

Another option may be to remove yourself from the source of the mold. This might mean moving or changing jobs.

Once that's done, you'll be able to remove the toxins from your body.

If you continue to be exposed, it's unlikely that you'll be able to rid yourself of the mycotoxins. Unfortunately, that can be difficult if your exposure is coming from somewhere that you don't control such as your workplace, your apartment, etc. Even if you do have some control, it can be expensive to have the mold source properly remediated. Still, it's necessary to stop the source of your exposure.

If you suspect mold exposure, I'd suggest reading the book by Dr. Ritchie C. Shoemaker called *Mold Warriors: Fighting America's Hidden Health Threat*.

Assuming you've taken away the exposure, it's time to remove the mycotoxins from your body. Without treatment, they'll just circulate in your body without end.

When removing the mycotoxins from your body, the challenge for those detoxing while having ulcerative colitis symptoms is that treatment includes taking binders orally. Binders absorb the mycotoxins and take them out of the body.

For example, binders can include the prescription medications Cholestyramine and Welchol, and natural binders such as charcoal or zeolite.

Unfortunately, I have found that when I've taken binders, it irritates my gut. This is true for me even after I healed from ulcerative colitis.

Some very gentle binders I was ultimately put on (after healing) that I tolerated well are Pectasol and Mycobind. These are non-prescription supplement type products. As I said, these were tolerable to my gut, though I didn't try them when I had active bleeding and ulcerative colitis symptoms. I used them well after I was healed.

A far infrared sauna is one way to help remove toxins without ingesting anything.

If you do test positive for mycotoxins, I'd strongly recommend finding a doctor knowledgeable about the protocol developed by Dr. Ritchie Shoemaker, MD. You can find his site here:

https://www.survivingmold.com/

On his site, there are listings of doctors who know his protocol. You can also access a wealth of information there.

CHAPTER 15: UNRAVELING THE STRESS-COLITIS CONNECTION

Over the years, the intricate interplay between stress and the exacerbation of ulcerative colitis symptoms has become a subject of increasing interest. While stress is not considered the root cause of ulcerative colitis, its impact on the disease is undeniable.

Stress and anxiety activate the body's "fight or flight" response, releasing hormones like cortisol and adrenaline. In individuals with ulcerative colitis, these responses can potentially exacerbate inflammation and lead to symptom flare-ups.

Naturally, lowering stress and finding peace can help this condition, and many others.

When I developed ulcerative colitis, my research led me to realize that if I could reduce stress, it could potentially help my condition. Yet, how was I supposed to calm down when I was in such pain, with such a horrible disease? I realized that freaking out was only going to make my health worse. I knew I had to somehow get peace in the middle of this storm.

I did many things to help myself calm down as much as possible. For me, throughout adulthood, there has been one main way to battle anxiety and stress. That's through faith in God.

Throughout my life I've tended to be anxious. Meditating for an hour a day didn't alleviate it. Relaxation exercises didn't make a dent. Positive thinking wasn't much help. In fact, I had practiced it as much as anyone could. For some time, I had been a teacher of New Age principles and practices. I taught these things for many years in a variety of settings, including a college and various resort spas. Ultimately, I felt that there was no real power behind any of it.

What really helped me was to come to know the God of the bible, to change my view of the world to match His, to develop a relationship with Him, and to learn to trust Him.

In Him, I discovered power, peace, and a lot of help through life's trials. Brought up as a religious Jew, I came to believe in Jesus (or Yeshua in Hebrew) in my early 30's. It wasn't an easy thing to do. My parents tried to have me kidnapped to "deprogram" me. That, thankfully, fell through, but they didn't speak with me for over 10 years.

However, my faith came after much research into the science, history, archeology, and prophecies of the bible. I couldn't deny what I saw. I decided it was real, that Jesus was who He said He was. I gave my life to Him. I had powerful, supernatural experiences that confirmed my faith. God helped me through the difficulties that came when I made my choice to follow Jesus.

Eventually my relationship with my family was restored. My parents passed, and I believe my mother and father are now with the Lord.

Over time, I learned that I needed a personal relationship with the God of the bible. This comes by prayer, study, worship and by experiencing his presence. Not by ritual or manmade rules. Attending church alone doesn't do it, though it can change your life when you attend a good church where they believe in the bible as the word of God and teach you to know Him for yourself.

I've heard it said that sitting in a garage doesn't make you a car. Well, sitting in Church doesn't make you a follower of Christ. The bible says that God is a rewarder of those who diligently seek Him. Personally, I want His rewards. Most of all, I want Him.

From the time I made the decision to follow Christ, the quality of my life was so different. I have profoundly experienced real power, comfort, love, direction, purpose and so much more from the Lord.

Despite having a strong faith in God (Father, Son and Holy Spirit), I found myself in this rather terrifying situation. I knew from experience that God would help me. He has taken me through some very difficult circumstances.

I sought God hard during this time. I took time to worship, pray and read the bible. I have experienced miracles in the past. I have felt and experienced His leadings on a daily basis. I knew He was the answer to this situation (and every situation).

During prayer time, I felt the Lord asking me to trust Him, once again. He reminded me that He'd always come through for me. In the bible, there's a scripture that I've relied on through the years. 1 Peter 5:7 (ASV) says:

> ***"Casting all your anxieties on him, because he careth for you."***

I sensed that He was asking me to trust that it would all work out because the Creator of the Universe cares about me (just as He cares about you).

In the bible, One of God's names is Jehova Rapha, The God who heals. I had seen many miraculous healings with others, and even experienced a couple myself.

Yet, before the ulcerative colitis started, I still had some severely disabling illnesses. I was still hoping for my complete miracle. As I sought Him for it, God had sustained me through the illnesses, but I was still hoping for the entire head to toe makeover.

I do believe that the bible teaches that healing is available for those in relationship with Christ. Scripturally, physical healing can be shown to be in His sacrifice/atonement for our sins, and so I continue to stand in faith for the entire healing.

While I preferred to receive a miraculous healing of ulcerative colitis, since it would have been much easier, I had the ability and drive to research and find natural and alternative health support. I attributed that ability to God. I was grateful that I was still alive by the grace of God, despite my complex and long-standing health issues. I attributed that fact to God as well.

So, once again, God was asking me to make a choice, and I chose to trust Him.

I'm not saying it was always easy, or that I didn't experience anxiety, but faith in God is what I always came back to. Trusting God gave me hope, joy and greater peace. I counted on His direction and help and received it. Over the years, I had learned how to be sensitive to the leadings of God, and it's always paid off. I had to trust that it would pay off again.

This hope helped me to battle anxiety. And ultimately, it worked out. I feel He led me to exactly what I needed to heal from ulcerative colitis.

So, in my opinion, the one way to peace is through drawing close to God.

Focus on What's Good

Part of the way I have found more peace in my life was to keep my focus on those things that would lift me up mentally, emotionally, spiritually, and finally, physically.

While going through the healing process, another scripture influenced me to choose peace over stress in my life. Philippians 4:8 (NIV) says:

> *"Finally, brothers and sisters, whatever is true, whatever is noble, whatever is right, whatever is pure, whatever is lovely, whatever is admirable – If anything is excellent or praiseworthy – think about such things."*

I decided, as much as possible, to focus on positive, uplifting things rather than those things that would create stressful reactions in my body.

For example, because I was weak and in pain, I spent a lot of time on the couch in front of the TV during these months. It was all I could do. Once I understood that I was to change my focus, I chose to stop watching anything that made me tense. I'm a big movie fan, and that meant that I needed to stop watching some of the movies I found appealing. Instead,

I watched feel good TV series and movies such as comedies, love stories, musicals, etc.

I chose to avoid watching the news for a while, at least until I healed. I spent a good deal of time researching ulcerative colitis, of course. I also spent time reading the bible, meditating on scripture, and in prayer and worship. Finally, I spoke aloud to my body, commanding it to heal in the name of Jesus, according to scripture. I focused on speaking faith filled words rather than fear or complaining words. For me, this paid off.

I also took time to walk back through my life to make sure I had forgiven everyone. The bible teaches that we must forgive because we were forgiven. Carrying bitterness has consequences and can block the ability to receive all of God's blessings. I prayed over anyone that came to mind, forgiving them and blessing them, as the bible directs.

Bitterness and resentment can contribute to chronic stress, activating the body's stress response. Persistent stress can lead to elevated levels of stress hormones, such as cortisol, which, when chronically elevated, contribute to a range of physical health issues. Chronic negative emotions have been associated with increased inflammation in the body. Conditions like irritable bowel syndrome (IBS) may be exacerbated by chronic negative emotions.

Sometimes, counseling can be a great idea if things aren't going well in your life. It's helpful to work with a trained professional who can help you come up with better ways to see things, and more effective ways to deal with stress and stressful situations. If you've got situations in your life causing you stress, or for which you haven't had solutions, consider counseling. Be very choosy about the counselor you pick though. They will influence you.

If you have ulcerative colitis, it may be time to take care of yourself, and to do those things that can bring healing. Taking care of your heart and mind can only have a positive influence on your health.

Do you want to know Jesus?

It's easy. He wants you in His life. The bible says that all have sinned. Our sins separate us from God. He loves you so much, that He suffered and died on the cross to take the penalty for your sins upon himself. When you accept this free gift and commit your life to Him, your sins are forgiven, and you can enter into a relationship with God.

If you're not ready to commit to Him, you may wish to ask Him to help you become ready. Ask Him to help you to know Him.

If you are ready, you might want to say a prayer like the following:

> Lord Jesus, I repent of my sins and surrender my life to you. I believe that Jesus Christ is the Son of God. That he died on the cross to take the penalty for my sins and rose again on the third day. I believe that in my heart and make confession with my mouth, that Jesus is my Savior and Lord. Wash me clean and come into my heart. Help me to draw close to you.

If you prayed either of these prayers, I suggest you find a church that's considered "full gospel". That means that they believe in the bible as "the word of God". That means they believe the bible was from God to us.

I would also suggest finding a church that believes in the baptism of the Holy Spirit, and that God still heals today. These types of churches are where I've seen the most miracles.

The bible says that when you draw close to Him, He will draw close to you. Growing in closeness to God has enriched my life in ways I can't express. Ultimately, it can change your life to get around people who have maturity in the things of God.

I'm a fan of science fiction, and I particularly love stories that have time travel in them. I've thought about what I would tell my young self if I could go back in time. The biggest and most important thing I could share is that Jesus is real, and He loves me. I would tell my young self to give my life to Him right away, no matter what it cost me. I would say to study the bible, befriend those who love Him, and draw close to Him all the days of my life. There could be nothing more important, and nothing can bring peace and healing as He can.

CHAPTER 16: SUPPLEMENTS: BRANDS, DOSAGES

For your convenience, the following are the supplements I took and the dosages I used.

Berberine:

Integrative Therapeutics Berberine 500 mg per capsule.

Dosage: 2 capsules 3 times a day.

This is more than the recommended dose on the bottle so always consult with your doctor before using it in this way. This can lower blood sugar so those who are diabetic should speak to their doctor.

Boswellia Serrata:

I've been using a product that unfortunately has been discontinued. It's called Ayur-Boswellia serrata by Douglas Laboratories. Once I run out, I'll have to replace it with something equivalent. There are several on the market. Just remember to choose one that's gluten and dairy free.

The product from Douglas Laboratories has

200 mg of Boswellia serrata Extract (Boswellia serrata, gum) standardized to 65% Boswellic Acids.

Dosage I used: 2 capsules, 3 times a day.

Collagen Powder

Clean and Happy Living Agglomerated Pure Hydrolyzed Collagen Peptides.

Dosage: 1-2 scoops a day.

As I mentioned, there are many of these on the market that are equally good. Stick to organic, grass fed, if possible.

Colloidal silver

Argentyn 23 Professional Bio-Active Silver Hydrosol 23 PPM.

Dosage: I started out on 1 tablespoon hourly and on the second day I went down to 4-5 times a day.

Argentyn 23 is known for its purity and small particle sizes. This makes it more easily absorbed and excreted. This product is used in some doctor's offices for intravenous use. I've had this as an IV on one occasion.

Digestive Enzymes:

Enzymedica – Digest Gold.

Dosage: I took 1-3 capsules each time I ate, depending on the quantity of food. If I ate a small meal, I would use one Digest Gold. If I ate more, I would take more capsules.

Enzymedica – Lypo Gold

Dosage: If a meal was fatty, I'd add 1 Lypo Gold to the Digest Gold capsules I was taking.

elete Electrolytes:

This is made by Mineral Resources International, Inc. (MRI).

Dosage: I took it as directed on the bottle, as needed while I was experiencing diarrhea, and during the colonoscopy prep.

Gastrazyme:

Gastrazyme is made by Biotics Research.

Dosage: The recommended dose on the bottle is 1 pill 3-4 times a day. I took more than the recommended amount. I found that taking 3-4 tablets 3 times a day made a big difference for me as far as pain levels. It does have vitamin A, so you don't want to overdose. Vitamin A is one of those vitamins that can cause problems if you take too much. I only used that dose for a short period of time – a few weeks. Still, I can't say that it's safe for everyone to do that. Again, since this is more than the recommended dose on the bottle, consult with your doctor before using it in this way, and consider having your vitamin A levels tested if you use this product in this way.

Goldenseal root:

Nature's Way - Premium Herbal Goldenseal Root - 570 mg per capsule.

Dosage: I was taking 2 capsules, 2-3 times a day.

This is more than the recommended dose on the bottle so always consult with your doctor before using it in this way.

This should not be taken long term as it can be hard on the liver. I personally don't usually take it more than a few weeks at a time.

Grapefruit seed extract:

Pure Encapsulations - Grapefruit Seed Extract

Dosage: I took 1 capsule 3 times a day.

L-Glutamine

Jarrow Formulas - vegan L-Glutamine.

Dosage: I took 15,000 mg of powder in water daily on an empty stomach. However, one doctor recommended taking that dose twice a day. Again, if you're dealing with cancer, I would skip this.

Magnesium

Target-Mins Magnesium Caps with silica by Country Life.

Dosage: As needed for constipation. I started low with one capsule and worked up until I got the desired effect. For me, that was usually 600 mg two times a day when constipated.

Manuka honey:

Manukora - UMF 20+/MGO 830+ Raw Manuka Honey

Dosage: I took ½ to 1 teaspoon while fasting, whenever hunger was a problem. That was probably about 5-10 times a day.

Some feel Australian manuka is the way to go, but this honey is from New Zealand. Having researched this brand, I felt it was good quality manuka and the pricing, though expensive, was a bit lower than some of the Australian honeys. It's gluten free, antibiotic free, glyphosate residue free, non-GMO and vegetarian. It's tested and traceable for authenticity. You can scan the code on the bottom of the bottle to see the lab results from your batch.

Olive leaf extract:

My personal favorite is a very expensive version called East Park Olive Leaf Extract Super Strength d-Lenolate 500 mg.

It's standardized with a patented process that creates a minimum of 18% oleuropein and as much as 23%. I've found it to be very effective over the years. I've tried other brands, but

I'm partial to this because it's worked. Still, if it's too expensive, I would purchase a more affordable brand.

Dosage: I took 2 capsules 3 times a day.

Probiotics:

Jarrow Formulas - Ideal Bowel Support - Lactobacillus plantarum 299v.

Dosage: I took 1 – 2 capsules a day.

Ultimate Probiotic (with a soil-based organism) by Silver Fern.

Dosage: I worked up to 6 capsules a day, and for several months, I took even more (as many as 12 capsules a day).

FMF (Functional Medicine Formulations) - Triple Therapy Probiotic Powder Sticks.

Dosage: I usually take 4 packets a day.

You can find it online here:

https://store.drruscio.com/products/triple-therapy-probiotic

Zinc-L-Carnosine

The brand is called Doctor's Best. The product is called PepZin GI Zinc-L-Carnosine Complex.

Dosage: I took 20 mg daily.

CHAPTER 17: WHAT DIDN'T WORK & ONE LAST THING TO CONSIDER

This will be a short chapter!

First, there were a couple things I tried that I don't feel helped.

Ozone Insufflation

I have a medical grade ozone unit that creates ozone gas for medical purposes. It can be used to make ozone water, or the gas can be used in the rectum, vagina, ears, etc. I have found it very healing and anti-inflammatory. I've used it for many years, though I hadn't used it rectally for quite some time.

I decided to try the gas inserted rectally, to see if it could help. I had found some research suggesting it might. I was still bleeding at the time.

Unfortunately, this made the bleeding worse. I stayed away from using the gas rectally for several years and have only recently started using it again that way, occasionally, with no problems.

Supplement IV's

For many years I've taken regular IV's of glutathione, and also high dose vitamin C. I'd usually get a 2000 mg glutathione IV once a week, and a 25,000 mg vitamin C IV once a week or every other week.

These have made a major difference for me in a variety of ways. I don't know where I'd be if I didn't have these IV's. However, although I increased the vitamin C IV's to almost every other day, they didn't seem to make a dent in the ulcerative colitis symptoms.

One Last Thing to Consider

Undetected and untreated infections anywhere in the body can cause the immune system to misfire. Whether it's bacterial such as with Lyme disease, or viral such as with the Epstein-Barr, it's important to identify them and deal with them.

In my experience, a hidden dental infection can wreak havoc on your body. It can cause all kinds of symptoms, and it's even dangerous. You'll be swimming against the tide if you're trying to heal while you have a hidden infection, including dental infection.

Your doctor can test you for the common varieties of viruses. Testing for Lyme disease can be tricky because of a high incidence of false negatives. IGeneX is a lab known for having better Lyme disease tests. If you suspect Lyme disease, find what's called a "Lyme Literate" doctor, referred to as an LLMD.

For dental health, consider finding what's called a biologic or holistic dentist. They can use advanced equipment to spot tooth infections. They can also check for cavitations which are cavities or holes in the jawbone where there are pockets of infection.

Even with all of the modern equipment, unfortunately it can still be hard to identify infected teeth and cavitations.

Also, it's common knowledge now that mercury fillings are unhealthy. And root canals are very controversial, believed by some to cause chronic infection that can lead to health problems. It's something to research and consider as you work on improving your health.

Gum infections can also contribute to problems in the gut. There is ongoing research exploring the potential links between oral health, specifically gum infections (periodontal disease), and systemic conditions, including inflammatory bowel diseases like ulcerative colitis. While the exact nature of the relationship is not fully understood, there is some evidence suggesting a possible connection between periodontal disease and inflammatory bowel diseases (IBD). It's essential to care for the teeth and gums.

An undetected bladder infection can cause issues. If you've been diagnosed with interstitial cystitis or you've had bladder symptoms with negative test results, consider requesting a special urine test. MicroGen DX is a lab that tests urine looking using something called qPCR + Next Generation Sequencing. They can see what most other labs don't.

Lastly, consider that there may be an association between covid and ulcerative colitis. Covid, even mild cases, has been known to cause autoimmune issues. So, my thinking is that it's possible that there's a relationship there. Long haul covid or vaccine injury could be considered and treated.

While formal studies for treatment are starting to get underway, the process can take many years. However, there are now doctors around the world trying out allopathic and integrative treatments on their patients, and it's worth looking into if you think having had covid or taken the vaccination may have something to do with your condition. Start your search checking out the term "Long Haul Covid". I suggest searching on the duckduckgo.com browser as you'll get better results.

MY HOPE FOR YOU!

I hope this book changes your life for the better! We pray that you're led to exactly what you need to recover completely. We wish you a life full of health and blessings!

If you have any questions or if you'd just like to keep up with any new information, consider joining our Facebook group currently called "Healing Ulcerative Colitis Naturally".

Here's the group address:

https://www.facebook.com/groups/healucnaturally/

Please LIKE our Facebook page here:

https://facebook.com/HealingUlcerativeColitisNaturally/

If this book helped you at all, please visit our Amazon.com web page to leave a review. It will help us be seen in the search engine, so others might find help!

ACKNOWLEDGEMENTS

From A. Ball: Thank you to my darling husband who has stood with me through thick and thin. You are God's greatest gift to me. You're precious and loved.

Thank you to Pastors Bob and Jan Sutton who prayed me through so much, including this illness, and prayed this book into existence. I'm always grateful for your support, love and friendship.

Thank you to my little tribe of prayer warriors – Dayle, Sophia, Alonia, Roger, Chuck and Wes. You are treasured friends/brothers and sisters in the Lord, who have continually prayed and cared for me. God has blessed me through each of you.

Dayle, you've put in so much overtime praying for me, and investing in our friendship – thank you my special friend! I adore you.

And thank you to Pastor Richard Risi, my spiritual dad who has been there for me whenever I needed him, along with his lovely wife and my dear friend, Patrice.

REFERENCES

CHAPTER 1

PubMed Central, Intestinal Stem Cell Development in the Neonatal Gut: Pathways Regulating Development and Relevance to Necrotizing Enterocolitis, published online February 3, 2021. Lluis Espinosa, Academic Editor. Accessed online 3/11/2024. https://www.ncbi.nlm.nih.gov/pmc/articles/PMC7913590/

CHAPTER 2

Mayo Clinic, 2022, Colonoscopy, accessed 11/29/2023, https://www.mayoclinic.org/tests-procedures/colonoscopy/about/pac-20393569

Mayo Clinic, 2022, Flexible Sigmoidoscopy, accessed 11/29/2023, https://www.mayoclinic.org/tests-procedures/flexible-sigmoidoscopy/about/pac-20394189

CHAPTER 3

MedlinePlus, 2023, Ulcerative Colitis, accessed 12/1/2023, https://medlineplus.gov/genetics/condition/ulcerative-colitis/#causes

Sponaugle Wellness Institute, Can Mold Toxicity Cause Ulcerative Colitis? Find Out Today. By Dlynch90. Copyright 2023. Accessed 12/1/2023, https://sponauglewellness.com/mold-toxicity/can-mold-toxicity-cause-ulcerative-colitis/

Celiac Disease Foundation, What is Celiac Disease?, accessed 12/27/2023, https://celiac.org/about-celiac-disease/what-is-celiac-disease/

Celiac Disease Foundation, Slowly Responsive Celiac Disease, accessed 12/27/2023, https://celiac.org/about-celiac-disease/poorly-responsive-celiac-disease/

CHAPTER 6

PubMed Central, 2021, Analysis Of The Anti-Inflammatory Capacity Of Bone Broth In A Murine Model Of Ulcerative Colitis, Amosy E M'koma, ACADEMIC EDITOR, ACCESSED 12/16/2023, https://www.ncbi.nlm.nih.gov/pmc/articles/pmc8618064

WebMD,Health Benefits of Gelatin, Medically reviewed by Dany P. Baby MD on February 6, 2023, Written by WebMD Editorial Contributors, accessed 12/24/2023, https://www.webmd.com/diet/health-benefits-gelatin

PubMed Central, Intermittent Fasting and Reduction of Inflammatory Response in a Patient with Ulcerative Colitis. Published online August 11, 2023. Ludovico Abenavoli, Academic Editor. Accessed 3/11/2023. https://www.ncbi.nlm.nih.gov/pmc/articles/PMC10456230/

CHAPTER 7

WebMD, Should You Try a Low-Residue Diet?, October 30, 2023, Medically reviewed by Brunilda Nazario, MD, accessed 12/25/2023, https://www.webmd.com/ibd-crohns-disease/crohns-disease/low-residue-diet-foods

The Paleo Mom, Dr. Sarah Ballantye, What is AIP?, accessed 12/25/2023, accessed 12/25/2023,https://www.thepaleomom.com/start-here/the-autoimmune-protocol/

Book: *Breaking the Viscous Cycle* by Elaine Gottschall B.A.,M.Sc., The Kirkton Press, Copyright 1986-2018.

Book: The Maker's Diet by Jordan S. Rubin, Destiny Image Publishers, Inc., Copyright 2004, 2005-Jordan S. Rubin.

CHAPTER 9

Book: Integrative Medicine (Fourth Edition), Chapter 50 (Inflammatory Bowel Disease) by Alyssa M. Parian, MD, Gerard E. Mullin, MD, Jost Langorst, MD, Amy C. Brown, PhD, 2018, accessed online 12/16/2023, https://www.sciencedirect.com/topics/immunology-and-microbiology/boswellia-serrata#:~:text=Gerhardt%20et%20al.,mesalamine%20for%20treatment%20of%20CD.

PubMed Central, 2017, The Roles of Glutamine in the Intestine and Its Implication in Intestinal Diseases by Min-Hyun

Kim and Hyeyoung Kim, accessed online 12-22-2023. https://www.ncbi.nlm.nih.gov/pmc/articles/PMC5454963/

Cleveland Clinic, 5/23/2022, Collagen, accessed 12/22/2023, https://my.clevelandclinic.org/health/articles/23089-collagen

CHAPTER 10

PubMed Central, 2003, Probiotics and inflammatory bowel disease, by Daisy Jonkers, PhD and Reinhold Stockbrugger, MD, accessed 12/23/2023, https://www.ncbi.nlm.nih.gov/pmc/articles/PMC539443/

CHAPTER 13

PubMed Central, Low Dose Naltrexone for Induction of Remission in Inflammatory Bowel Disease Patients, March 9 2018, Mitchell R. K. L. Lie, Janine van der Giessen, Gwenny M. Fuhler, Alison de Lima, Maikel P. Peppelenbosch, Cokkie van der Ent, and C. Janneke van der Woude, Accessed 2-10-2024 on: https://www.ncbi.nlm.nih.gov/pmc/articles/PMC5845217/

CHAPTER 12

PubMed Central, Article called Examining the Effects of Glyphosate Exposure on the Gut Bacteriome and Inflammation in a Murine Model of Colitis. Published online February 26, 2020, Authored by J A Barnett, N Haskey, C S Quin, R Bonnie, A La Berge, A Ale jandra Verdugo Meza, M

Hart, and D L Gibson. Accessed 2-10-2024 on: https://www.ncbi.nlm.nih.gov/pmc/articles/PMC7043650/#:~:text=Conclusions,in%20Muc2%2D%2F%2D%20deficient%20animals.

Glyphosate Toxicity Alert: How American's #1 Weedkiller Tricks Your Body Into Absorbing It, Written by Isaac Eliaz, MD, MS, Lac, July 16, 2020, accessed on 2/10/2024, https://draxe.com/health/glyphosate-toxicity/

PubMed, Integrative medicine and the role of modified citrus pectin/alginates in heavy metal chelation and detoxification. Written by Isaac Eliaz, Elaine Weil, Barry Wilk, December 12, 2007. Accessed 2-10-2024 on: https://pubmed.ncbi.nlm.nih.gov/18219211

YOUR NOTES

This is where you write down anything you'd like to remember, to do, or to research further.

Medical Tests I want to take:

Supplements I'm interested in taking:

Supplement Name	Dosage	Times per day

Strategies to take on:

Things to research or consider:

Made in United States
North Haven, CT
13 October 2024

58887356R00098